EAT
to CHEAT
AGING

What you eat helps make 60 'the new 50' and 80 'the new 70'

by dietitian, Ngaire Hobbins
APD, BSc., Dip. Nutrition and Diet

First published in 2014

PO Box 478

Northbridge NSW 2063

AUSTRALIA

Text © Ngaire Hobbins

Illustrations © Reg Lynch

Not to be copied in whole or in part without written authorization.

ISBN 978-0-9943440-0-7

Printed in Australia through Book Production Solutions

Contents

Introduction

Ngaire Hobbins is a leading nutritionist specializing in nutritional care of older people right up to the frail elderly. I have had the pleasure of working with Ngaire in my multi-disciplinary team at Brisbane Waters Private Hospital in New South Wales.

Nutrition for older age groups is not a favored topic in the popular magazines and too many people believe they can still diet or eat in the same way they did when they were much younger. As Ngaire points out, optimal nutritional care in older age is paramount to prevent complications of malnutrition including falls, confusion, infection, rapid decline and premature death.

Ngaire sets-up a real challenge for us to extinguish the previous incorrect stereotypes of the nutritional requirements for both fit and frail elderly and expel the myth that as you get older you need to eat less.

Ngaire highlights that too many frail older people are on inappropriate and highly restrictive diets which contribute to sub-clinical starvation. They should in fact be *avoiding* low fat foods and consuming the exact opposite of what we all thought, even higher fat and higher calorie foods, to maintain adequate calorie, protein intake and maintain weight.

Nutritional care of the elderly is generally poorly managed, under recognized, under diagnosed and under treated. With the advent of specialized medicine and the "single organ approach" to patients' medical problems, their nutrition is unfortunately rated low on the priority list.

Ngaire notes that malnutrition is a major risk factor for ill health in the elderly and is a major contributor to post-operative complications in a hospital setting. Poor nutritional care results in otherwise preventable hospital admissions, a prolonged and expensive hospital admission with many potential life threatening complications. It is in the interest of all hospitals to elevate nutritional care as the cornerstone of health care for all patients including the elderly.

In my clinical experience as a Consultant Geriatrician I commonly see frail elderly people with multiple co-morbidities including dementia, Parkinson's disease, stroke, heart disease, gait and balance disorders who have associated severe malnutrition.

Malnutrition rates are up to 80 percent in elderly living in hostels and nursing home, and at least 50 percent of community-living elderly over the age of 80 have some form of malnutrition.

Ngaire's book is a very practical approach to identify the risk factors for malnutrition and offers easy strategies to eliminate those risks and improve nutrition and health for everyone facing older age.

I once said that it is a paradox of modern medicine that doctors pay little attention to the nutritional care of the elderly when it is so common, produces catastrophic complications yet is easily preventable.

This book will improve the health of many elderly people and I hope it keeps them more active and more independent for longer.

DR PETER S LIPSKI
MB BS MD (Syd) FRACP FANZSGM
Consultant Physician in Geriatric Medicine
Director of Geriatric Medicine – Brisbane Waters Private Hospital
Conjoint Associate Professor Newcastle University

Chapter 1

USE IT OR LOSE IT

The hidden roles of the muscles and bones in your life

Muscle: the anti-aging frontline

Did you know the key to living long and living healthy lies in more than merely avoiding illness, it lies mostly with your muscles?

It's true. They do a lot more than move you around — they hold the keys to cheating aging. And they are more vulnerable than you might imagine.

You may have managed to keep up the gym work, the cycling, swimming or whatever is your thing, and secretly gloat over how athletic you look or — if your muscles are now hidden by an extra bit of padding you've stacked on — how well you've been able to disguise your more generous shape. But no matter what's obvious on the surface or how you might feel, the unseen changes caused by age, wear and tear, illness and stress can rob you of muscle minute by minute.

Why is that important?

Muscle does so much more for you than you may realize. It helps maintain every one of your body's organs, helps you avoid type 2 diabetes, and ensures your brain is adequately fueled to coordinate all that activity and keep your mind firing as you'd like it to. It keeps blood coursing in your veins, oxygen moving through your body and food being processed to supply fuel and nutrients. It also helps you fight illness and infection and is essential for repair work that ranges from healing everyday bumps and bruises through to tissue, bone and tendon repair after major surgery.

Unfortunately, the effects of muscle loss can become nothing less than disastrous if you remain blissfully unaware of its significance and don't work to head off any loss.

Medical advances may have managed to conquer illnesses which once claimed lives at a younger age, but making the most of the extra 20 years or so most of us have gained as a result depends on you finding ways to keep your body (especially your muscles) and brain going a lot longer than our grandparents might have needed to in their lifetimes.

Generations ago, eating of course meant hunting and gathering, and that meant running, climbing, throwing, digging, carrying really heavy stuff like whole animals, and walking, walking, walking. If you wanted to eat, you had no choice but to keep your muscles working.

Sure, the hunter–gatherer lifestyle is no longer a career option, but unfortunately we humans are way too good at finding ways to do less and less activity, and that's not only bad news for our muscles but ultimately for our immune system, body organs and our brains.

I for one don't wish to return to my grandparents' days of scrubbing floors on hands and knees, walking miles to work every day, and living without my mod cons. But even if these bygone lives seemed hard, they worked body muscle as it needed to be worked.

My grandfather was born in the early 1900s. In those days 65 was considered quite a ripe old age — time to retire on the old age pension and potter around the house. Nowadays 65 is positively young and it's not for nothing that 60 is considered the new 50. People expect far more from their remaining years than the generations before did. You want to be able to travel, to get down and dirty with the grandkids, to embrace new technology — Skype, Facebook, perhaps online dating — and maybe even take up belly dancing or skydiving.

Grandad had to chop and split wood and carry it up to the house every day just to get a cup of tea in the morning. He had to push a hand-mower across the lawn each Saturday and, if something had to be repaired, out came the hammer, the handsaw, the hand-drill and the manual screwdriver. Today we push a button to boil the jug, push a button to start the mower which almost drives itself and we can't imagine life without the electric drill, the chainsaw and perhaps even the electric nail gun.

My grandmother did her washing in the copper, dragging each item out of the scalding water with a stick and putting it all through a hand-wringer that strenuously objected if the sheets dared bunch up too much. The wringer then had to be released, the washing unwound from around the rollers, and the whole process started again. Then the still very wet and very heavy load had to be carried out to the washing line. The line was a floppy wire strung across the yard and propped up with long poles that needed to be angled low when grandma pegged out the washing, then re-angled to hoist the washing higher to avoid dogs and small children playing as the washing dried (try doing that with a heavy load of wet washing on the line). She was judged by her good housekeeping and religiously mopped the floors and dragged the carpets bodily out of the house, draped them over the back fence then beat the dust out of them with a cane carpet beater. She even made cakes as light as air using only a wooden spoon, a hand-beater and elbow grease.

It's ironic how we've become so clever in thinking up an endless array of gadgets and machines to do so many physical activities that we've outpaced

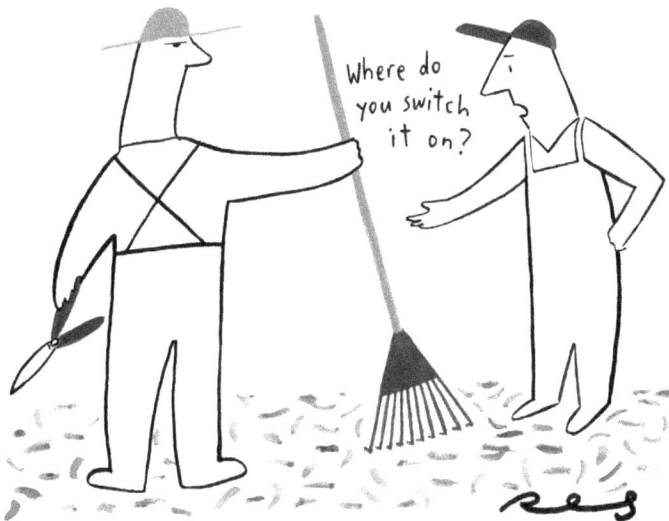

the way our body systems evolved over time. And yet they still depend on us to keep functioning well and keep going about their work. I need to go to the gym to achieve the sort of strength and muscle grandma took for granted.

And the older you get, the more important muscle becomes.

It's fortunate that there is a lot you can do to keep your muscles up to scratch. Understanding what your muscles need is pivotal, and with that, understanding the role of what you eat.

None of us want to give up our TV remotes, our washing machines or our electric drills, so we need to find *alternative* ways to keep the life in our muscles before it's too late. That not only means staying active and doing exercise which boosts muscle but you also need to feed them right, and that's about changing focus from,

eating to avoid illness, to eating to 'cheat' aging.

Most well-worn health messages aim to get us to avoid the big health baddies like heart disease, but those messages just don't have the same relevance when you get older. Of course they're still important, but it's time to change emphasis. The message is not to ignore eating advice on how to help avoid heart disease or other preventable illnesses, but it's about realizing that things are different when you look ahead beyond your 60s. Because, as you reach your 50s and 60s, it's also about cheating your body into effectively thwarting what its physiology — the body's processing and functioning — naturally inclines it to do, and that's to gradually slow down.

Slowing down physiology-wise means that body systems won't work as well as they once did. But your muscles are able to help you out if you help them. Sure some 'rust' will set in anyway and illness can take a toll, but your muscles and what you eat and do to support them can head off age-related decline. That will give you power to make the most of the 20 or 30 or so years ahead.

To look more closely at how easily the wheels can fall off, consider **Joan and Betty:**

Joan and Betty did most things together in life. There was golf, a bit of tennis, plenty of socializing and getting out and about with friends and families. Joan had always been just a bit more active and seemed always to have been able to eat yet stay thin, while Betty had struggled to keep her weight down for most of her life.

Both slowed down a bit from their mid 50s, but not enough to cause any concern. Life was good and they felt they'd earned a chance to rest up a bit. But, as Joan did less she also found herself feeling less hungry and her meals became smaller. She was conscious of maintaining her health and read up on various diets. The one that appealed was to eat mostly fruits, salads, vegetables and wholegrain foods with just occasional meat and fish and some low fat dairy foods.

Her friend Betty just enjoyed her food too much to cut down. She tried to share her friend's interest in her diet and managed to go along with it some of the time too, though not always with the same determination or success.

When Joan lost some weight she wasn't worried. She felt quite virtuous. Betty didn't lose any but didn't gain either; so felt she was doing okay.

By 68 they both felt well and were living good, healthy lives.

Now this all seems perfectly reasonable and appropriately healthy right?

Wrong. In fact there are a couple of red flags in this picture that may surprise you: weight loss, eating smaller meals and eating fewer high protein foods.

Joan was well intentioned, but the diet she chose was for her younger self, and not the best plan for the years ahead of her. Age imposes unique nutritional needs no matter how well you eat and what you weigh. Losing weight once you are older, means losing muscle and that sets you up for poor health ahead. And those smaller meals, along with less meat and dairy foods mean fewer essentials — like protein — to help you cheat aging.

This is still the time to review and realign your ideal food choices, even for those of you who are more like Betty. Although Betty felt so far from Joan's lack of interest in food and her ability to gradually lose weight that she may as well have inhabited another planet, surprisingly, of the two, Betty was in fact the better off when it came to staying independent and healthy into *the future. That 'healthy' diet you might have been trying hard to stick with may no longer be right for you. We'll come back to the girls soon.*

Eating and working to maintain muscle in your later years will help you fight infection, quickly and efficiently repair any injury you suffer — big or small — keep your brain cells firing and of course preserve that spring in your step.

Why muscle is more to you than merely what moves you.

Your muscles are your reserve supply of body protein.

Why is that important? Protein is constantly being used to do the body's repair work. Every little thing your body has to do every minute of every day means wear and tear on your cells. And every cell in every organ — in your skin, your gut, your blood, and all the substances running the systems that keep you alive — has a lifespan. Some have only hours of life, some days, some months before they are replaced with new ones. Protein is used minute by minute for this constant renewal. And at the same time it's helping fight off infection and fueling your brain — we'll get back to those later in the chapter.

You eat food, and food contains protein so what's the problem?

It's rather like your car. Once you turn that key, you expect to be able to travel many kilometers. Your car needs fuel to keep running but you don't carry the petrol station (or the power point if you have entered the brave new world of electric cars) around with you for that constant supply. Your car's fuel tank is your reserve between fill ups and muscle is our protein reserve between food fill ups. But unlike our cars, which we can switch off when the day's work is done, there is always a need for protein somewhere in your body, day and night — even when you are sleeping — so the protein fuel tank (your muscles), is always in use.

Protein is released from your muscles to bridge any gaps between food fill ups. And those gaps come along surprisingly often: they include the non-eating hours between meals; the times if you are unwell when you just can't eat properly; or if you fast — for medical, religious or other reasons — and there are always days when, somehow, you just don't get time to eat the meals you should.

In a car you start with a full tank, travelling along at whatever pace you choose and if you don't refuel a time will come when you will just stop abruptly. It's different for your body — it's not all or nothing. If your protein reserve dwindles enough, all those systems which rely on it can start to falter and you face more of a slow, grinding halt.

Fortunately, even those of us who don't look like Mr or Ms Universe are blessed with a start-up muscle supply that far exceeds what's needed. And that's important because muscle, unlike your car's fuel tank, has so much to do beyond being a protein reserve. It's obvious that muscle keeps you moving about but it also helps you avoid type 2 diabetes (or manage it if you already have it) and that is an important asset in cheating aging, as you will learn in Chapter 6.

Holding onto the muscle you have, boosting it if needed and replenishing it as much as possible if any is lost will always keep plenty of protein in reserve when you need it.

Back to Joan and Betty:

Around comes the cold and flu season and Joan succumbs. And you know what it's like with the flu, you don't always feel like eating. Joan's muscle reserve is furiously releasing protein to augment what little food she feels able to eat. Her immune system is able to rage along on the protein reserves supplied by her muscles while food isn't available to do the job, and Joan recovers. But in the process she has lost some muscle (along with a bit more weight). So what happens now?

For things to reset to how they were before the illness, Joan needs to replace the muscle (and protein reserve) she has lost, not to mention the weight loss prior to that. Betty is in a better position, not having already lost some weight. It's Joan who is the concern here because this is where age raises its somewhat unattractive head. It's harder to rebuild muscle the older you get. Not just because exercise becomes less and less appealing to most, but also because of the ageist bias of our physiology.

MUSCLE IS NEEDED TO:

- stop you from falling if you should lose balance or miss your step
- allow you to keep exercising effectively and moving around safely
- support your joints to reduce the pain of arthritis and similar conditions and maintain your flexibility
- support the function of your heart and lungs
- help you to continue to swallow safely and effectively
- help boost your appetite
- help your body use insulin effectively to avoid diabetes developing or worsening
- keep fuel supplied to your brain
- help you avoid having an adverse reaction to a medication

So, move the muscles that move you!

Those raging hormones were not all about sex after all

In your younger years, adopting that Adonis look was, if not exactly effortless, certainly more feasible. Bodies growing into healthy adulthood are hard-wired to build muscle. And if any was lost while your muscle reserve was temporarily doing its rescue work, you were conveniently programmed to rebuild it as soon as you ate again.

But that programmed rebuilding requires a combination of three things:

messages from hormones

signals from nerves

the activity of muscles themselves.

And here's where our bodies' ageist physiology strikes again. Hormone levels diminish and the signals from nerves dwindle with age. From as early as your 30s or 40s both are affected and, by your mid 60s, hormone and nerve boosting of muscle has all but ceased.

That leaves muscle *activity* alone in the rebuilding task. But, your muscles are reminded to repair and build *only* when you work them. Fortunately, even though it gets more difficult to completely rebuild the older you get, that system does keep working into your later years.

So if your body is to have any chance at all of keeping pace with the plans you've made for the years ahead, it needs your help.

Those flabby arms and bingo wings, flibberty bits, saggy bottoms and turkey necks might be gravity's joke but under that exterior it's up to you to nurture your inner Adonis.

That means considering five things:

1. Eating for your muscles: getting enough protein

Ironically, after all those years when most of us seemed to struggle to keep our meal sizes within civilized boundaries, when we were often being told to eat less meat and dairy and that the pinnacle of good nutrition was a plate piled to the ceiling with salad and veggies topped with nothing but a squeeze of lemon, the time has now come when a lot of that will get turned on its head. Not everyone is going to find themselves eating less and less food as they get older, but improbable as it seems, very many of us will. And while all those lovely vegetables, fruits and leafy things provide irreplaceable vitamin and antioxidant boosters, the meats and cheeses of this world take on an elevated status from now on.

Why? Because you are still running an adult-sized body no matter how old you are and it still has adult-sized needs for most nutrients. In fact, with all the extra wear and tear amassed as the years pile up, you need *more* of some things than you did when you were younger — and protein is one — so the importance of packing extra nutrition into your meals to keep your muscles up to scratch and cheat aging is undeniable. You don't have to eat huge amounts of those protein foods but you mustn't eat less than you did when younger. And many of us will need extra protein.

Chapter 4 will guide you on *how much* protein there is in foods, the choices to make in different situations, plus ways to ensure adequate protein intake if you are vegetarian. (See the following list of protein foods.)

But life is too short to spend on having to think about every mouthful you take. So make it easy on yourself:

Just put a protein food at the center of most meals from now on and you won't have to struggle to get what you need.

When you ate larger meals you could easily get away with having protein foods only at some meals or in very small amounts as a 'garnish' while vegetables, fruits and grains held center stage. In fact that's the ideal diet plan to combat obesity in younger people and is what you will often hear or read is right for older as well as younger adults. But, unless you include a good protein food at most meals you risk not being able to cope with your body's demand. And, don't forget, if you do suffer an illness or an infection you will need to eat even more protein to help balance what your muscles will lose. That means eating protein between meals and, for many, adding high protein drinks or supplements.

GOOD SOURCES OF PROTEIN

All meats, fish, poultry and seafoods	all fresh cuts or processed — including ham, bacon, smoked meat, poultry and sausages and all products containing red meat, poultry and fish.
Dairy foods	including milk, cheese, yoghurt (but excluding cream and butter) also milks, cheeses and yoghurt from goats and sheeps
Soy products	including soy milk, yoghurt, tofu, tempeh and others
Pulses	including lentils, chick peas, dried beans and peas
All nuts and seeds	and products made from them
Wholegrains	and products made from them

2. Animal vs vegetable protein

Let's face it, if you need more protein than years ago but don't want to eat bigger meals or if you are finding yourself eating less than you once did, then it stands to reason you need to pack more protein and other essentials into every serve.

That means animal foods have the advantage because your serves of meat, fish, egg or dairy food don't need to be as large to get the same amount of protein as they do when it comes from most plant foods (such as soy milk, nuts, seeds and grains).

We also know from sports science that animal protein is able to help build muscles in athletes more than most plant proteins can, especially if it's eaten close to the time when you exercise (ideally within an hour). Building and maintaining muscle is of course of immense importance to athletes, but even if you are not planning to run a four-minute mile any day soon, your muscles will still benefit in the same way.

Years ago, concerns about fat and cholesterol may have had you eating less meat, eggs and dairy but those concerns don't stack up the same way now. Protein is now so very important and the other nutrients those foods supply are a bonus. Low fat diets, too, are no longer what most of us need now. It's time to ditch those concerns of our youth and enjoy one of the benefits of reaching a mature age!

And while it's always best to get protein from meals so you also get the benefit of the nutrients in the accompanying foods, occasionally you might need to add high protein drinks (see the recipes in Chapter 8) or use a commercial protein supplement. The array of supplements in the supermarket aisles can be bewildering but those based on the dairy product, whey (whey protein isolate or whey protein concentrate), are considered to do the best job. If you are vegan or vegetarian you might prefer formulas based on soy protein isolate.

You are not going to achieve a Charles Atlas body, or whoever his svelte female counterpart might be, but supplements might just give you the boost your muscles need at times when you are not able to get a good serve of protein at each meal (and in between meals if you need the extra if you are ill or recovering from illness).

PROTEIN CONTENT IN FOODS AND THEIR EFFECTIVENESS IN PROMOTING MUSCLE GROWTH

Food type (listed in order of the general ability of the protein they contain to boost muscle growth)	The amount of food needed for 20 to 30g protein per meal (listed for each food)
Whey protein isolate powder	20g (approx. 1 dessertspoon)
Meat or fish (cooked)	100g (size of a regular pack of cards or 1 small tin of tuna or salmon)
Skim milk powder	60g powder (approx. 2 tablespoons or 600ml liquid skim milk)
Egg	3 eggs
Milk	600ml (or approx. 80g or 3 dessertspoons milk powder)
Cottage cheese	140g
Cheese (cheddar or similar)	3 slices of processed cheese or equivalent sized amount
Yoghurt	400g (large tub)
Soy protein isolate powder	20g (approx. 1 dessertspoon)
Soy milk	900ml
Lentils	400g can
Almonds	about 95 nuts or 130g (1 cup)
Tofu	200g (about the size of 2 packs of cards)
Rice (cooked)	6 cups
Bread (sliced)	9 slices

3. Muscles are forgetful and need memory jogs

Like you and me, muscles like to be reminded they're needed. There's no getting round the saying, 'use it or lose it'. Sure it's harder to keep your muscles the way they were, but unless you keep using them, and using them well, they'll forget what they're there for.

That means you need to think about the type of muscle activity you do. First of all, there's the benefit of gravity. Our muscles thrive on the effects of gravity and you can use that to your advantage by avoiding sitting or lying down too much. Of course you need to rest but don't get complacent: keep looking for ways that gravity can help you every day: get up, stand tall, move around, carry things, use the stairs, park further from the shop, walk instead of drive, rake the lawn, sweep the floor. There are endless examples.

And then there is exercise itself. Sadly it's just not enough anymore to stroll around the shops or to go for a leisurely walk. In order to boost muscle function at every chance, you need to do activities that stress your muscles and help make up for those absent hormones and vastly diminished nerve triggers.

And because you have muscles everywhere, it has to be activity that works not only your legs, but also your upper body, arms and abdomen. Your muscles need to work against a weight (called resistance exercise) to encourage them to build. Luckily, 'resistance' doesn't only mean lifting weights in a gym. Aquarobic exercise or swimming laps uses the water as resistance. Walking briskly or uphill, sweeping or raking the leaves instead of waving the leaf blower about, taking the stairs more often, even doing supervised exercises like tai chi or 'over 50s' fitness classes are all good as long as they get your heart rate up and have you puffing and sweating a little. (There is a list of suggested activities to maintain your muscles below.)

All these activities need to be checked with your doctor first of course and carefully supervised as you get older, but that doesn't mean you shouldn't do them. Accepting age as a reason to do less and less physical activity, to sit most of the day and to have lots of daytime naps, as too many do, will only do you harm in the long run.

And as soon as you are able after an illness or after being immobilized for any time, you will need to work extra hard to help recover what you might have lost. It may not be what you feel like doing, but it will certainly help you out when you are faced with any similar challenges. (See the extra suggestions for recovery below.)

Joan and Betty were wrong to believe that what Joan had read in magazines and diet books applied to them, and they were wrong to believe that slowing down and eating less was 'just a part of getting older'.

The rules about what is good for you now you are older are not the same as those which applied when you were younger. If you could count on living only until your late 60s, your muscle reserves may well hold out without much help. But as you are likely to live well past those years, your health and independence in the future depends on those reserves still being there when you need them in your 80s and beyond. And that won't happen without you making an effort.

EXERCISE GUIDELINES FOR RECOVERY AFTER ILLNESS OR IMMOBILIZATION

Resistance exercise is the most important for recovery. Don't expect it to increase the size of your muscles as that's unlikely, but it will help in your recovery, boost your strength and ability and improve your longer term health.

You can start with either no weights, or very light ones, but add extra when you can, or do extra repetitions on the same weight so you progress in strength.

As soon as you are able — even while you are confined to bed (and as long as it's safe to do so) — start to do as much as you can even if it's only one or two activities at first.

Work up to doing 8 to 12 repetitions of exercises for each major muscle group: legs, arms, abdomen, hips, back, chest, shoulders.

If you have had surgery or an injury and are in hospital, check what you are able to do with the physiotherapist or ask your doctor.

As soon as you are able, return to doing all your maintenance activities.

GUIDELINES FOR EXERCISE TO HELP MAINTAIN MUSCLE FUNCTION

The ideal is to combine aerobic, resistance, flexibility and balance activities, so you need to find activities which you are able to do, which don't put you at risk of falling and ideally which interest you. Professional assistance is ideal but not essential. Everyday activities like vacuuming and mopping, raking, sweeping, gardening, carrying the shopping and doing housework also contribute but adopting the following are your best bet to cheat aging:

Aerobic

- on at least 3 days per week initially, increasing to every day
- aim for 30 to 60 minutes each day, which can be accumulated in 10 minute bouts
- make at least 20 or 30 minutes of this time at vigorous intensity (puffing and sweating)

Resistance

- weight training on at least 2 days per week
- exercises for all major muscle groups: legs, arms, abdomen, hips, back, chest, shoulders
- repeat each exercise 8 to 12 times
- increase the weight you lift as it gets easier or repeat more times

Flexibility

- sustained stretches for each major muscle group on at least 2 days per week
- use static stretches, not those involving movement

Balance

- on at least 1 day and eventually up to 7 days do 4 to 10 different balance activities in a safe environment only, repeat each 1 or 2 times
- There is more detailed information including examples of exercises and how to measure your exercise intensity in the appendix of this book.

4. For your muscles, being bed-ridden is like being in outerspace

Being immobilized through illness — also somewhat misleadingly called 'bed rest' — is more harmful to your muscles than merely leading an inactive life. It affects your body in much the same way as being in zero gravity for an astronaut, and the more so the older you get. Lying around robs you of muscle and once you are older it doesn't come back automatically.

If you have had an accident, surgery or sickness, chances are you will spend some time in bed and during that time your muscles won't get their usual workout. And that workout includes the everyday fight against gravity to keep you upright as well as everything else you do to remind your muscles what they are there for. So, although you may not feel like doing anything more active than eating delightful hospital cuisine and drinking stewed tea while you are confined to bed, you are going to lose muscle if you don't get up as soon as you can or at least do some exercise while you are there.

There is a silver lining: some of the lost muscle becomes protein reserve and is diverted into repairing wounds, combating infection or fighting off fever.

But unfortunately, the combined losses through diversion into repair work and the lack of exercise can be very large. Realizing what's going on and working to minimize the effects can be your key to stopping a vicious cycle of muscle loss and illness which then could potentially trigger increasing frailty and chronic ill health. Get active as soon as you are able, so that muscle loss won't become permanent.

Be clear, you might also lose *body fat* with any of this type of weight loss, but that's not the bonus you might think it is because weight loss during immobilization, illness or after surgery is a sign all-important muscle has certainly also been lost.

If the time in bed is only a day or two there's little to be worried about, enjoy the rest. But over a period of 10 days or so, it can easily rob you of 1kg of body muscle — a lot to lose. (See the next page for a perspective on muscle loss.)

Daytime rests can also be an issue if they get out of hand. A nanna nap can certainly be replenishing, but too much rest time *every* day just means your muscles are missing out.

HOW MUCH MUSCLE DO I HAVE AND HOW CAN LOSING IT AFFECT ME?

The amount of muscle we have varies enormously depending on how much resistance exercise we do regularly. For most moderately active people in the healthy weight range muscle is usually about 40 percent of bodyweight.

- muscle loss increases your chance of gaining excess weight and your likelihood of developing type 2 diabetes or hampering management if you already have diabetes
- during a major illness, losing just five percent of body muscle reduces the function of your internal organs and slows wound healing
- with a loss of around 20 percent of body muscle, organs begin to fail
- death can result from a 40 percent loss of body muscle.

For an older person weighing between 65 and 70kg, you could easily lose five percent of your body muscle by losing 5kg of bodyweight.

5. The problem of an over-enthusiastic immune system

Your immune system is able to rally the 'protein troops' to mount a defence almost the instant a foreign substance enters the body. It's working before you're even aware you've been invaded, and it can neutralize a threat before any symptoms get the chance to appear.

It's an awesome response plan and it efficiently protects you from illness. Your muscle releases protein to be converted into specialized immune substances as soon as the system starts up and keeps doing so as long as it's active. But, as you age, the system can become overactive so that your muscles release protein to the immune system more often, or for longer than they should. Small amounts of muscle can continue to be lost even when you have recovered or are feeling quite well — often over quite long periods of time. Sometimes your immune system can also react when there is no real threat and that's a big problem for your muscles because targeting unwanted invaders uses muscle protein.

You won't always know it's happening, though weight loss might be a tell-tale sign. But you should always assume that you need to actively rebuild your muscle reserves after any illness now that you are older.

The same recovery strategies you need to put in place after immobilization will also help head off any lingering losses after illness.

How did Joan and Betty go you ask?

Well, in true happy ending tradition, they got great advice, both revved up their activity levels, started to eat more good-protein foods and felt so much better that they took up pole dancing at 70! (Well, no, that's just a rumor — as far as we know — but they did go on a cruise and kicked up their heels!)

It's easy and mostly common sense to avoid muscle loss setting you up for ill health, but so many people inadvertently make choices that don't help. Muscle can be lost for many years before stick-thin arms and legs make it physically obvious and, all the while, the body's systems, which rely on that muscle protein reserve, can be faltering. It's hard to reverse if it goes on too long: avoidance is so much easier.

All this talk of eating more seems to fly in the face of what you may read about eating plans which restrict food intake to boost health benefits. But these plans are not things you should suddenly take up if you are closer to 90 than 50 for good reason: read why in Chapter 5.

How to help your bones remain strong

Does it surprise you to know that bone is not a static structure? It is constantly being remodeled much the same as muscle.

Bone has a soft protein framework made hard when minerals — calcium (mostly) and phosphate — are added to it, making a dense, strong structure.

It's also a stored reserve of calcium which, among other things, is needed by your heart to keep it functioning properly. Did you know that if you don't eat enough calcium for both your bones and your heart, the extra that your heart needs will be robbed from your bones?

Bone builds when there is adequate protein, calcium and vitamin D available and when signals from hormones and active muscles 'tell it' to rebuild. Bone's constant rebuilding and remodeling keeps it strong and dense as long as replacement = removal.

After middle age any losses from your bones aren't always replaced, and bone density can fall, making bones weak and vulnerable to fracture.

Trips and stones may break your bones

Consider Frank.

Frank was never a big person and prided himself on his slim build. He was fiercely independent and after his wife died he was determined to cope alone in his own home 'until the end'. He was not a big exerciser at any time in his life: he played bowls after he retired and busied himself at home and in the garden but had a gardener to do the heavier work.

Since his mid 60s he had very gradually lost weight and by the time he reached his late 70s was quite thin. But he took no medications and continued to do most things he wanted to, just more slowly, and was insulted by the suggestion made by his doctor on one rare visit that he should consider a stick or other walking aid as well as further assistance at home.

But then disaster struck. One day while putting out the bin, Frank stumbled on the path and fell against the low brick front fence. He suffered a fractured hip and a number of nasty grazes and bruises.

In hospital he was found to have osteoporosis and was vitamin D deficient. Frank was surprised. Osteoporosis was something his wife had worried about but he didn't think it would affect him. And he never thought that his careful avoidance of the sun could do him any harm.

Unfortunately Frank's story isn't as hopeful as Joan's. His reduced muscle reserve along with the osteoporosis slowed his recovery after surgery and when he did return home, he needed a lot of assistance to stay there.

Could Frank have avoided his sudden loss of independence?

Certainly accidents happen, but a lot could have been done to minimize the impact of his fall so he could still be happily living completely independently. Osteoporosis can affect men as well as women if you don't remain active and eat to support your bones.

It's no surprise to anyone that breaking a bone is bad news, but at later age it's not only bad news, it's a potential disaster. First there's the immobilization while you recover — which further robs you of both bone and muscle — then the added physical assault of surgery should it be necessary (not to mention the far higher risk of complications, wound infection and even death in surgery for older people), and of course the knock to your confidence and ability to move around as you did before.

Having strong bones won't stop you falling but it might help you avoid a fracture if you do.

OSTEOPOROSIS

Osteoporosis is the extreme of low bone density. It is the cause of one person being hospitalized with a fracture every hour of every day!

In Australia one in every two women and one in every three men over 60 are likely to suffer a fracture due to osteoporosis.

Osteoporotic bone, when viewed on an x-ray, appears to be filled with holes and becomes extremely fragile. Your chances of developing it are higher if you:

- have a family history of osteoporosis
- don't get enough exercise
- you smoke or drink excessive amounts of alcohol
- you don't get enough calcium and vitamin D
- have certain illnesses including rheumatoid arthritis
- take certain medications for long periods of time, including steroids

There are many organizations providing excellent advice on avoiding and dealing with osteoporosis, and some contact details are listed in the appendix of this book.

If you have already been diagnosed with osteoporosis there are things you can do to keep as much strength in your bones as possible, and maybe to even add some. There are medical treatments and the same food rules apply whether you have osteoporosis or not. Exercise is important but check with your doctor and/or your physiotherapist before you embark because you may need a carefully designed plan to avoid causing damage.

Food for your bones

Calcium is what gives bone its strength. Protein forms the framework and helps absorb the calcium from foods, and vitamin D is essential for that calcium to be incorporated into the bone. You need all three to keep your bones up to scratch.

All of these are covered in greater detail in Chapter 4, but vitamin D warrants special mention. Most of what we get naturally is made in your skin when it's exposed to the sun, but skin cancer risk has reduced people's sun exposure.

As vitamin D is scarce in most foods (with the exception of a few — including oily fish like salmon, natural butter and some foods, like margarine, to which it has been added), a vitamin D supplement, or a mixture of calcium and vitamin D are often prescribed by doctors and dietitians to assist your bone density.

I read somewhere that eating lots of protein causes calcium to be removed from your bones. Is that true?

This was a concern a few years ago but it relates to research in younger people eating very large amounts of protein foods with limited calcium.

It's not a problem in older people.

Protein foods instead boost the absorption of calcium so that makes those foods useful as you get older. Getting both protein and calcium is important. Of course dairy foods supply calcium along with protein and even some vitamin D and they don't need to be low fat now you are older. And full cream dairy foods might even be easier for the body to use.

Exercise for your bones

Exercise and activity are not just for your muscles, they are just as important to your bones because as muscles work to move your limbs and body around, they cause the bones nearby to flex just a little. This sends 'signals' which help boost bone density and strength.

Your bones, as much as your muscles, pay a high price for the declining activity levels and limited hard muscle workout that our modern lives provide. Everyday activities of life — moving round your home or the shops — won't help your bones sufficiently once you get into your later years. They need exercises which 'stress' them more than that. Fortunately, the same exercises that are good for your muscles also help your bones. (Take another look at the lists of activities for your muscles in this chapter and in the appendix.)

To 'stress' those bones a bit in everyday life:

- walk up stairs instead of using the lift
- walk faster rather than slowly
- use ankle or hand weights when you exercise.

Resistance exercise (lifting or pushing a weight with your arms, legs or whole body) and weight-bearing exercise (the type in which you actually carry your body weight) are the keys. If muscle weakens, so will bone, if you are immobilized, bone is also lost. If you don't eat enough to maintain your weight, your bones will lose out too.

Medications to help your bones

There are a number of medications that can help boost your bone density and reduce osteoporosis. In fact, in later age, many medications do a lot more to help your bones than diet alone can do. But it's important to be aware that these medications must be taken strictly as directed. Some that have been around for a while require you to take a tablet soon after waking, and then to sit upright for around half an hour before you eat or drink anything. If you lie down during that time or if you eat too soon, the medication can irritate your esophagus (the tube between your mouth and stomach, also called the 'gullet') and eventually make it uncomfortable or difficult for you to swallow food.

Newer medications to preserve bone don't have such requirements: check with your doctor and follow the directions carefully on any you have been prescribed.

Chapter 2

USE IT OR LOSE IT

Ways to keep your brain active and healthy and help stave off Sneaky AL

Everything that applies to your muscles also holds true for your brain: keep it active and feed it properly.

An active brain means you'll be able to continue to engage in spirited conversation, prepare and savor great meals, enjoy music and books, decide if a piece of art is worth the canvas it's painted on, plan and accomplish every day-to-day task, judge the safety and appropriateness of everything you do whether it's walking along a beach or doing the shopping to driving a car or playing tennis, and will allow you to keep on track with the people and the world around you.

Keeping all that up and fending off Sneaky AL (Alzheimer's) is more than doing sudoku or learning Russian. All those games of tennis, yoga classes, long beach walks, hours at the gym or whatever you do to keep physically active also help boost your brain by keeping up a good flow of both blood and nerve signals.

Eating the right food, coupled with keeping physically active and mentally stimulated, not only keeps up fuel and nourishment, it's critical to protect your highly vulnerable brain cells from damage which could otherwise lead to cognitive decline and Alzheimer's or other forms of dementia.

One likely suspect in the mystery of what causes dementia is the long term effect of damage to brain cells. That can happen as the result of fairly obviously traumatic incidents like accidents or an injury to your head, but it can also be anything that starves your brain cells of blood and/or oxygen (like strokes or the effects of high blood pressure and cardiac disease).

Amazingly, sometimes our brains are able to adapt, 'reassigning' tasks that damaged cells would otherwise undertake, so you get to continue as usual for many years.

What's less obvious, and a far more common issue that can't benefit from reassigning tasks, is the cumulative effect of years and years of tiny amounts of damage resulting from the everyday wear and tear of life. Every one of your body cells achieves what it has to by using a process called oxidation. Oxidation is absolutely essential to life, but it also results in some by-products (that you might know as 'free radicals' or oxidants), which can be harmful if they are allowed to build up. And this is especially important in your brain because more oxidation happens there than in any other organ in your body.

While each individual bit of damage probably has as much effect on your brain as a single drop of water has into an ocean, if allowed to accumulate, eventually your brain's ability can be swamped.

That's where eating comes in. Food contains antioxidants that mop up and neutralize free radicals before they can wreak havoc. So the more antioxidants you eat, the better chance you give your brain (as well as the rest of your body).

But more on antioxidants later.

First a look at what cognitive decline is all about:

Dementia? Memory lapse? Cognitive decline? Or Alzheimer's?

Before you write off lapses in memory as dementia or Alzheimer's, be aware that poor memory, periods of confusion or even altered behavior do not always mean dementia has set in or is even close. There is a lot you can still do to help your brain if you're experiencing these problems.

First and foremost, don't delay in discussing any concerns with your GP or geriatrician. It's understandable to be anxious about receiving a diagnosis you don't want, but memory lapses and confusion can also be caused by completely treatable conditions. If you put off mentioning these concerns to your doctor you could miss your chance of having something treatable dealt with quickly so you can get back to enjoying life.

And, if you did have dementia, the medications that are available to slow its progress, tend to be more effective if taken early, so don't ignore your concerns.

Is it dementia or just a temporary memory lapse?

Increasing forgetfulness doesn't necessarily mean dementia, and quite often your memory can still improve. Everyone has occasions when they can't remember where they've left the car keys, or 'why did I walk into this room, what was I going to do?' moments.

Forgetfulness might even be a blessing; after all, if you remembered every person you met and every tiny thing that happened to you in your life, it would drive you crazy!

But a little beyond forgetfulness is what's called cognitive decline or mild cognitive impairment. The word 'cognition' covers all the 'thinking' processes of the brain: coordinating things like memory, language (both understanding it and speaking), insight and judgment, problem solving, and decision-making. It's when some or all of these abilities permanently decrease that it becomes distressing.

Mild cognitive decline is when you consistently forget things such as appointments or important events, lose your train of thought, find it difficult to follow the plot in movies or books, feel overwhelmed by making decisions and make increasingly poor judgments.

It can be annoying but it doesn't overly interfere with your everyday life. It might show up on tests and be obvious to you and to others who know you well, but it's usually manageable and doesn't always progress further. If you do regular exercise — both physical and mental — and eat appropriately it can even improve.

But, unfortunately, mild cognitive decline for up to 20 percent of people will move on to dementia in time.

How does dementia or Alzheimer's disease differ from cognitive decline?

Dementia (including Alzheimer's disease which is a type of dementia) is **not** a normal part of the aging process and cognitive decline is only part of the picture.

Dementia interferes with your everyday life and, therefore, often the lives of those around you. Everyone is different, but the sorts of things it throws up include not being able to learn or remember new information, repeating stories and questions over and over, having difficulty finding words for familiar things, jumbling words and phrases, losing or hiding possessions, forgetting how or when to do everyday activities, becoming agitated and confused and even suffering hallucinations.

Dementia is a progressive and fatal illness. It may have only minimal effect for up to five years in some people but then can progress quite quickly. Some people live up to 20 years after they have developed dementia, but most live only 10 to 14 years.

A word of caution here. Other things can masquerade as dementia. Don't confuse it with what may be delirium or a deficiency of vitamin B12. Some of the same traits you see gradually revealing themselves in dementia — confusion, agitation, disorientation, incoherent speech, hallucinations and extremes of emotion — can also be caused by either of these. But there's a very big difference. Unlike dementia, delirium and B12 deficiency are curable, so their symptoms will go away once they are dealt with.

Delirium

Delirium is a serious, life threatening medical condition that can occur when you have an infection, experience fever, after a general anesthetic, when you are dehydrated, and in a number of illnesses.

It's red herrings like confusion, disorientation and hallucinations that can make diagnosis unclear at times. A delirium might look just like dementia to the casual observer — it's easy to suspect it as the culprit when there's no obvious illness or fever — but there is an important clue to diagnosing it:

delirium usually comes on quickly and the symptoms can come and go, even with a day or so in between at times, though usually more pronounced at night. Dementia, in contrast, usually develops gradually over weeks, months or years and, once evident, symptoms tend to be constant.

You'd think it would be obvious if a delirium were due to an infection or similar because there'd be pain or fever but if you are already taking medication to control pain, the tell-tale signs can easily be masked.

Surprisingly, too, you can have infections bubbling away deep under your teeth, in your urinary tract, or even in your lungs, which actually cause no pain or obvious illness to alert you to their presence.

It's also quite possible to be unaware you are dehydrated and that in itself may be a potential cause of delirium.

And in yet another annoying reality, the older you get, the more likely you are to suffer a delirium during an illness, particularly if you regularly take more than four different medications of any kind, or if you have Parkinson's disease, already have dementia or have previously had a stroke. And if it happens once, there is a high chance, unfortunately, that it will happen again.

One thing to keep in mind, too, is that medications themselves can cause delirium: you may not tolerate a new medication prescribed for you, or you might accidentally take more of one than you should. Sometimes there is an interaction between different medications and sometimes you may have done well on a particular dosage level for many years but changes in the way your body deals with it as you age mean side effects can surface. One of those can be delirium.

The take-out message is that any sudden change in someone's usual behavior needs a visit to the doctor. And before you even think about changing anything yourself: **you must *not* stop taking any prescribed medication** without first discussing any concerns you have with your doctor. The sudden change itself might trigger delirium or cause other health issues. Have a look at the list in the box on the following page. If you have any concerns, your doctor can organize a thorough review of your medications — something that should always be done anyway if you have experienced delirium.

Delirium can also be a sign of other undiagnosed problems that need treatment to stop them doing more damage. If you do suffer delirium there's also more chance your illness will put you in hospital so, unless you are planning *that* relaxing experience, it's best to consult your doctor quickly.

SOME OF THE MEDICATIONS THAT MAY TRIGGER DELIRIUM IN OLDER AGE

*NOTE: **DO NOT STOP** TAKING MEDICATIONS PRESCRIBED FOR YOU WITHOUT CHECKING FIRST WITH YOUR DOCTOR. DOING SO COULD CAUSE SERIOUS HARM.*

All medications are prescribed for specific reasons and most people don't have any problem with them or, if they do, the side effects should quickly diminish. With advancing age and increasing medical issues, problems may occur with some medications on this list. If you are concerned at all for yourself or someone you care for, then discuss your options with your doctor as soon as possible. The list is only a guide and includes common brand names. Generic brands of some medications and those released recently may not be listed here.

Common brand names are shown in italics

Heart medications:	**digoxin** (*Lanoxin*) and **disopyramide** (*Rythmodan*) — both anti-arrhythmia drugs; **isosorbide** (*Isordil, Isogen, Imdur, Monodur, Sorbidin, Iimtrate*) for angina
Blood pressure drugs:	**nifedipine** (Adalat, Adapine, Nifecard, Adefin). This medication is also used for angina and Raynaud's disease
Anti Parkinson's medications:	**levodopa** (*Madopar, Sinemet, Kinson*)
Fluid tablets:	**frusemide** (*Lasix, Urex*)
Sedatives:	**barbiturates** (phenobarbitone, amylobarbitone)
	benzodiazepines (including *Xanax, Kalma, Valium, Serepax, Ativan, Diazepam, Rivotril, Murelax*)
	alcohol

Anti epileptic or anti-psychotic medications:	**phenytoin** (*Dilantin*)
Some antidepressants:	**lithium** (*Lithicarb, Quilonium*), **SSRIs** (including *Zoloft, Aropax, Cipramil, Lexapro, Prozac, Lovan*) and **TCAs** (including *Tryptanol, Allegron, Endep, Tolerade, Tofranil*)
Opioids (for strong pain):	**codeine** (marketed as *Codeine,* also *Aspalgin, Codis, Codral, Codalgin, Mersyndol,* and in many cold and flu medications), **morphine** (*Anamorph, MS Contin, MS Mono, Kapanol*), **oxycodone** (*Endone, Oxynorm, Oxycontin*), tramadol (*Tramal*) and **pethidine** (*Parnate, Nardil*)
Some **NSAIDS** (for pain and inflammation):	including **ibuprophen** (*Nurofen* and many generics) and naproxen (*Naprosyn*), available 'over the counter' and a number of common prescription NSAIDs:, **diclofenac** (*Voltaren*), **celecoxib** (*Celebrex*), **meloxicam** (*Mobic*), **piroxicam** (*Feldene*), **indomethacin** (*Indocid*), **mefanamic** acid (*Ponstan*)
Some anti-ulcer drugs:	**cimetidine** (*Tagamet*)
The anti-inflammatory corticosteroid:	**Prednisone** (*Delta-cortef, Panafcortelone, Solone, Premix, Sterofrin, Prednefrin forte, Panafcort, Sone, Medrol*)
Antihistamine:	**promethazine** (*Phenergan, Painstop syrup, Prothazine, Panquil, Seda-quell, Avomine, Tixylix*). These are older type antihistamines — the ones that also tend to cause drowsiness.
Some antibiotics:	**quinolones** (including *Ciproxin, Avelox, Noroxin*) **penicillin**-related drugs **amoxycillin** (including *Amoxil, Moxacin, Cilamox, Alphamox, Fisamox, Augmentin, Clavulin*) and **flucloxacillin** (including *Floxapen, Flopen, Flucil, Staphylex*), the **cephalosporins** (including *Keflex, Ceporex, Ibilex, Ceclor, Keflor*)

Note: Medication brand names will vary depending on the country of purchase.

A **deficiency of vitamin B12** also causes confusion and memory problems and it's something that can be too easily mistaken for dementia. But B12 deficiency is easily detected with a simple blood test and then is completely reversible if treated promptly. Delaying treatment, on the other hand, can cause permanent damage to your brain and nervous system.

B12 deficiency and its causes are dealt with later in this chapter.

Keep eating to keep your brain protected

It may seem improbable but the day will likely arrive when your appetite will not constantly persuade you to make the most of every morsel that comes your way. You may skip meals or just not think about eating. Whatever the cause, the mere routine of eating three or more meals a day is especially important to your brain as you age — for two main reasons:

The eating habit

The first is that eating is a habit thing and that means you can also get in the habit of missing meals and then you'll struggle to get enough nutrients for your brain and your body.

If your appetite has decreased, have a look at Chapter 3 where problems with appetite and how to deal with them are covered in more detail.

Glucose is the fuel for your brain

The second reason why eating is so important for your brain is because it uses different fuels to most of your body and it's very demanding!

Even though your brain is only about two percent of your body weight, it's so metabolically active (a medical term for being really 'busy') it uses up a whopping 20 percent or more of your body's total energy supply. Keeping up with demand requires a dedicated fuel supply system, with constant access to the blood sugar, glucose. This is in contrast to the rest of the body which can use stored fat easily as an alternate fuel if glucose runs low.

The glucose the brain needs comes from carbohydrates in food and from the limited amount of carbs stored in your muscles and liver. But this supply can run down very quickly — in less than a day if you are not eating well. If faced with the possibility of running short of glucose, your brain takes command, pulls rank and sends instructions to convert protein from the large reserve in your muscles into glucose so it doesn't miss out. That means it gets glucose where it can by converting other body reserves — and since body fat *cannot* be used to make glucose for the brain, but protein can, the reserve used will again be your muscles.

Keeping up your food supply — especially carbs and protein — will help you stay in the eating habit and stop your brain draining your muscle reserve. Eating to supply both brain fuel and muscle reserves is absolutely vital.

POINTERS TO KEEPING YOUR BRAIN GOING

1. Keep eating!

2. Fuel your brain

3. Keep your fluids up

4. Eat colours (and as many different foods as you can)

5. Keep exercising and remain socially active

6. Challenge your brain with puzzles, reading, crosswords and similar, learn new things and keep up with what's happening in the world

7. From now on don't become too thin. That little bit of extra fat around your middle may be good for the brain!

8. Be vigilant for any unintentional weight loss, and don't let it continue

9. As far as brain nutrients go, these are the heroes you need to watch:

    omega-3s

    the antioxidant vitamins: A, C and E

    the B vitamins: niacin folate, B6 and B12

    iron, zinc, selenium

    vitamin D

Fluids are your brain-lubricants

Your brain just can't fire on all cylinders if you are even a little dehydrated and, if dehydration worsens, it can present the brain with almost insurmountable challenges, bringing on confusion and incoherence all too easily. If you are unwell, dehydration also makes delirium more likely, not to mention that it hampers the work of your kidneys and worsens a whole lot of conditions that affect older people.

And even when you know all this, good hydration can still be a challenge when you get older because you don't tend to feel thirsty as soon as you should.

Something you might not know is that a lot of the water our bodies need each day comes from the food we eat. Some comes from the water content within food, but some also comes from the digestive process as foods are broken down. So, not eating well makes dehydration even more likely.

Diuretics

Some medications also contribute to dehydration, especially diuretics (commonly called fluid tablets) which are designed to remove excess fluid from your body to relieve some of the symptoms of heart problems. Keeping a balance between too much fluid affecting your heart and having enough to keep the rest of your body functioning is something that needs close monitoring by your doctor. Your medication needs can vary with weight loss and changes in your health so don't assume you always need to stay on the same dose of diuretic medication. As with any issue about medications, be sure to discuss any concerns you have with your doctor.

Water

Most people should have between six to eight glasses or cups of liquid each day. Ideally that would be water but almost any drink or even liquid meals will work.

(Sorry, but alcoholic drinks and very strong coffee don't provide as much fluid as you may like to think, so don't rely on them.)

If you are eating quite well and haven't lost weight then you probably don't need the extra energy (kilojoules) that juices, soft drinks, milk etc. supply. Water is the best option.

If you have lost some weight or are struggling to eat well, then by all means choose those extra kilojoule drinks (in moderation) as well as flavored milk, protein shakes and smoothies to boost your energy and nutrient-intake along with your fluids.

A drink with each meal as well as something between meals should give you enough water. Just be careful if you like to drink tea with your meals because it can affect how well you absorb some nutrients from the food in those meals. Read more on this in the discussion on iron in Chapter 4 but, if possible, it's best to enjoy tea between meals.

If you are really struggling to eat, don't fill up on water before a meal if it's going to mean you won't feel like eating the food you need.

Eat colors: the antioxidants for your brain

Think of the damage that free radicals or oxidants can do to your cells as somewhat like rust damage to iron. You might even be able to imagine it physically encrusting your cells when those joints creak and groan, but in the brain that 'crusting' is often unnoticeable until it's well advanced. That's where antioxidants become invaluable: they are a bit like anti-rust for your cells.

Antioxidants, and related food components go by a mystifying assortment of chemical names and some are also vitamins and essential minerals but, in a delightfully convenient twist of nature, many really beneficial ones also happen to come from colorful foods. So you really don't need to know much about nutrition to make sure you get plenty of antioxidants, you just need to eat a variety of colors. Ideally, eat at least five or six different colored foods, or shades of color at each meal, more if you can manage it. And no, that doesn't include five different shades of donut icing or colored sprinkles, it means natural coloring in real foods!

Many intensely colored foods are well known sources of antioxidants: think berries, cherries, red apples, egg yolk, dark green vegetables, green herbs, black olives, multi-colored lettuce, black and green tea, turmeric and other spices and the wide array of colored fruits and vegetables, not to mention dark chocolate. But even paler foods like green and gold apples (both the flesh and the skin), nuts, fish and mushrooms are good sources. You don't need much of each.

It's when the *variety* of foods you eat dwindles that your antioxidant intake also falls. With fewer antioxidants available to mop up free radicals, damage to brain cells gets more and more likely as the years go on.

As a result, it's tempting to look towards the almost endless variety of commercial antioxidant supplements, drinks and tablets on the market. But antioxidants may not work as well alone as they do when they are in the food they originally came from. There are other substances in the same foods that help out in ways we are only just starting to understand and no doubt more will be known of these in the next few years. What's important is realizing that they are sociable little fellows, much happier working with the team they already know. We just can't be sure they are as effective when expected to work independently. Eating as many different colored foods as possible is likely to be far more useful.

(You'll find a list of foods to eat to get different antioxidants in Chapter 4.)

Live life to the full — for your brain's sake

Exercise, social activity and mental challenges are more than just enjoying life and learning.
Keeping up an active lifestyle, exercising and eating well are good for your muscles and bones *and* good for your brain.

Physical exercise of course keeps blood flowing through the brain, but its benefits go beyond that. Keeping up the coordination of all the different systems involved — working your muscles, your balance systems, all the senses needed to see, hear, feel and plan those activities — also exercises your brain. If you do physical exercise regularly — sufficient for your muscles to work hard enough so that you feel it — you help your brain do better in other things and stem cognitive decline.

Not surprisingly, your brain also likes to learn and to be challenged by new things. So when you learn something you haven't done before — an exercise program like tai chi perhaps, new card games, different crafts, new skills or languages or when you make the effort to meet new people or practise skills that require concentration like crosswords or calculating in your head — all are doing something more for you than filling in your days. They're reminding the brain it's needed and can even cause it to form new internal connections to keep up the pace.

What's often not recognized is that keeping up social activities is really beneficial. Hanging out with other people means much more to the brain than merely avoiding loneliness, it means it must continue to mastermind all the very complex thought processes involved in making conversation, behaving appropriately, negotiating, and all the other things you need to juggle in social situations.

In fact, even without doing mental exercises, it's the people who keep up social involvement along with physical exercise who have the best brain health. The healthiest and longest-lived older people are those who have been active throughout their lives and continue to be so into their later years.

The added bonus of remaining socially involved, from a food point of view, is that doing things socially often includes meals or, at the very least, snacks!

Don't get too thin — what's that all about?

Throughout this book, everything about keeping active and eating to avoid unintentional weight loss, applies to your brain too. But I'm sure you'll be delighted to hear that it seems a bit of extra padding in later age can help your brain function.

Among the wide range of shapes and sizes you see in older people, on average, it's those who are a bit heavier who seem to have the advantage (at the higher end of the weight charts with a Body Mass Index or BMI, around 25 or even a bit higher). They tend to have better brain function and live longer than those who are much thinner (at the lower end of the chart with a BMI below 22).

Who knows why this is; maybe those who are heavier are that way because they have been eating more food and getting the benefit of extra nutrients. It could also be because, perhaps surprisingly, fat actually *does* something other than just boost cuddliness. Body fat cells produce very small amounts of hormones that might help protect brain function once you are older. So, when body fat is lost, so is that protection.

Whatever the reason, if you are already in your late 60s or older, the message is clear: if you are just a bit cuddly, it's probably not a bad thing for your brain. Dieting to lose weight now will do more harm than good (as discussed in Chapter 5).

In contrast, exercise (as discussed in the previous chapter) will do plenty of good even if it doesn't result in weight loss. It will help your heart, your joints *and* your brain and will help head off damage due to diabetes.

But don't for a minute imagine that obesity or overweight in younger people is good, it's not!

In fact, if you are still in your early 60s, your 50s or younger and are significantly overweight you are at higher risk of dementia as well as other obesity-related illnesses. Fortunately, you still have time to get your exercise levels up to boost muscle, lose fat and help your brain before it's too late.

For those heading into their 70s and beyond who have always been lean, don't rush out to try to gain weight. Just stop listening to advice suitable for 30 and 40 year olds that suggests a BMI around 20 is ideal —science begs to differ for you now. And, instead, gaining a few kilos could even be your best advice.

Special mention needs to be made about type 2 diabetes, often associated with being overweight, and which does seem to increase your chance of developing dementia. Science doesn't yet know exactly why this is so, but the theory is that this somehow makes the brain become less responsive to insulin in some people resulting in changes within brain tissue that contribute to Alzheimer's disease. Those who have been inactive and overweight throughout their younger adulthood and middle age, or who already have type 2 diabetes are especially at risk. Fortunately though exercise continues to help, no matter what weight you are. Combine that with eating to help your brain and you'll get the most benefit. (Read more on diabetes in Chapter 6.)

But what about very lean, fit older people?

Of course this is the ideal. There are plenty of examples of fit, lean, older people with excellent mind powers. Being leaner is no disadvantage as long as you remain very active and eat appropriately for your age.

But you do need to be extra vigilant about any weight loss. Without the buffer of a bit of extra weight, lean people lose muscle very quickly if they are ill or confined to bed for any reason, and of course that becomes a fast track to physical and mental decline.

As long as you keep up the exercise, continue to eat a good variety of foods including the protein you need, and don't lose weight, your brain and body will benefit.

Brain nutrients

An outline of the nutrients you especially need to watch now you are older, where to get them, how they work and how some interact with medications is covered in Chapter 4. Here's just a brief mention of those that are especially important to your cognition or brain function.

NUTRIENTS ESSENTIAL TO PEAK BRAIN FUNCTION

Glucose for brain fuel:

Fatty acids and micro-nutrients for protection and function:

    omega-3 fatty acids

The vitamins:

    B3 (niacin), B6, B12, folate and vitamin D

The minerals:

    iron, zinc and selenium

The antioxidant vitamins:

    particularly vitamins A, C and E

Omega-3 fatty acids (fish oil and similar)

Omega-3 fatty acids (going also by the abbreviations ALA, EPA and DHA) have been in the media over and over in recent years because of their benefits to both heart and brain.

Many generations ago these unsaturated fats were once much more common in the foods we ate. You can still get them from oily fish, wild or game meats, meat and milk from animals which eat grass rather than grain, as well as from some nuts and seeds and from the oil made from them. But a large amount of the food we eat contains little or none, or has other oil and food components that reduce how much we get.

Because of that, omega-3 supplements (including fish oil, krill oil, flaxseed oil) are extraordinarily popular. They are mostly extracted from high omega-3 plant seeds and marine animals such as very small ocean fish and krill (the very small sea creatures eaten by whales).

There has been quite a bit of research done looking at omega-3 and that continues. Many scientists suggest taking high doses of omega-3. But common sense is important: it's tempting to think that if omega-3 fatty acids are obviously important to the brain, and that our modern diets don't readily supply them, then taking as much as possible in supplement form will always be good. But, like everything, a balance is prudent. Omega-3s are also contributors to oxidation reactions in cells — they help brain function — but free radicals are produced in the process so antioxidant substances are important to counterbalance their effect. In contrast, taking high strength supplements or a small pile of omega-3 capsules without the benefit of those other nutrients in real food might not be as helpful as you might hope.

If you do choose to supplement what you get from food by taking omega-3 as fish or krill oil, keep in mind that it can take many, many kilograms of small fish or krill from the ocean to make just one kilogram of the oil in those tablets, so be sure you are not taking more than you really need.

FOOD SOURCES FOR OMEGA-3 FATS

ALA	flax seeds (linseed)
	walnuts
	leafy green vegetables
	some oils, particularly canola
EPA and DHA	fish oil
(also called long chain omega-3s)	fish and other seafood, especially oily cold water fish like salmon, tuna, mackerel and sardines
	grass fed meats and poultry
	wild meats (like kangaroo or rabbit)
	egg yolks
	the brain and liver of meat animals

A lot has been written about DHA especially (from fish and krill oil). It's found in high levels in the brain and is absolutely essential to protect brain cells from damage, but it's most likely that all omega-3s have important roles to play — which medical research has not yet completely identified — and relying on only one type may miss some benefits the others can provide. ALA it seems, may help your brain cells keep up fuel supplies, and EPA looks like it may limit the production of substances that contribute to Alzheimer's disease.

As is the case with most things in nutrition, variety is probably the key to heading off cognitive decline as well. If you don't eat many of the foods in the list here, a moderate dose supplement may well be something you could consider. But do also be aware that omega-3s can affect the action of some medications so always tell your doctor if you are thinking of taking these supplements.

An interesting thought is that, if seafood or fish oils were the complete answer, then vegans, who eat no EPA or DHA, and many vegetarians who get very little, would suffer faster cognitive decline and that's just not the case. There has to be something we are not yet aware of beyond these omega-3 fats alone.

The widely touted Mediterranean diet may well gain its plusses from the abundance of antioxidants it supplies from fruits, vegetables and good quality olive oil along with the omega-3 and good protein from fish and seafood.

The B vitamins

Folate

A deficiency of folate (also in foods as 'folic acid') is well known to cause cognitive decline. When levels of this vitamin are low in your body your chances of developing Alzheimer's disease are significantly increased.

Luckily folate is found in a lot of foods and if you eat well you'll usually be okay. Problems can crop up because some common medications interfere with the way folate is used in the body. Chapter 4 lists these medications for you. If you take any of these medications for more than a week or so you *should be having your folate status checked regularly by your doctor* and may need supplements or other interventions if your levels are too low.

Take care though: don't take a folate supplement unless your doctor prescribes it. This is one vitamin you mustn't get too much of because it can worsen kidney problems or hide the signs of a damaging vitamin B12 deficiency.

Vitamin B12

Vitamin B12 is needed to make red blood cells and to maintain healthy nerves and if you are deficient you'll see confusion, reduced concentration and memory loss — all easily mistaken for dementia. Luckily, prompt diagnosis and treatment can reverse all of these quickly so it's important to check with your doctor if you are worried. It would be a tragedy if permanent nerve or brain damage happens when it could have been avoided.

As with folate, most people should easily get enough B12 in their diet, but vegetarians or those who eat limited amounts of animal foods might struggle. Again, this is discussed further in Chapter 4 but some medications have an effect on B12 absorption, and as you age it gets harder to extract B12 from your food. Unfortunately, B12 deficiency is quite common in older people so it's one to be especially aware of.

Vitamin B3 (niacin)

Niacin, along with the other B group vitamins (thiamine B1 and riboflavin B2) are needed to make chemicals which communicate between brain cells. There are lots of claims around giving niacin wonder nutrient status for the brain and, more traditionally, for heart function. Unfortunately, many are inflated claims. Vitamin B3 is certainly essential to brain function and in some people is used therapeutically to assist in managing heart disease but only under strict medical supervision to avoid an excess causing other problems.

Although it's important to be sure to get enough B3, a deficiency is rare unless you have been eating poorly for quite some time, and then it will be only one of many nutrients lacking.

Vitamin B6

B6 is important in assisting brain activity, but it also plays an integral part in regulating levels of a substance called homocysteine. You can read more on this in Chapter 4 but scientists have found that if we accumulate too much it seems to affect cognition as well as heart health. In fact, B6 has recently been touted as helping to avoid Alzheimer's disease, partly because of this ability.

As with the other B vitamins of special importance to your brain, B6 is in lots of foods so the chances you'll miss out are similar to niacin. So, as long as you eat many of the foods already identified as being good for your brain because of their antioxidant levels — including wholegrain breads and cereal foods, potatoes, nuts and seeds, meats, organ meats and fish, banana and avocado — you'll also have B6 covered.

Vitamin D

Much has been written about this vitamin in Chapter 1 and you will read more later in the book. Vitamin D is immensely important throughout your body and no less so in the brain where even a marginal deficiency is thought to contribute to depression as well as reduced cognitive ability.

Iron

Most people know that you become anemic if your iron levels fall too low, but what you may not know is that a mild iron deficiency, which isn't even obvious without a blood test, can cause cognitive decline.

Iron supplies indispensable oxygen to brain cells and, because the brain has so very many things going on, even a minor shortfall means it can't function properly. If that shortfall continues, permanent damage happens.

Iron is needed to make substances that convey messages between brain and nerve cells and also helps in their protection.

Three things can set you up for iron deficiency. Firstly, medical conditions which cause you to lose blood (e.g. from chronic ulcers in your stomach or upper intestine, anything which causes blood loss from the bowel — including bowel cancer—bleeding gums, or frequent cuts, bruises and grazes). Secondly, any medical issue or medication that reduces your ability to absorb iron from food. Lastly, but certainly not least because it's so very common, gradually cutting down on eating high iron foods like red meat.

It can take many months or years for your iron levels to get low enough to cause even a mild deficiency but if any of the above are familiar to you, make sure you have regular blood tests.

Prevention is, as always, prudent. From now on make sure you get high iron foods most days: liver (lambs fry), kidney, red meats, poultry and fish are the best sources so vegetarians especially should be vigilant.

Zinc

Zinc and iron are minerals found in the highest quantities in the brain, and people who don't get enough zinc suffer from reduced memory, learning ability and cognition. But get too much and it seems it might play a part in the development of dementia.

Too much zinc is something you would only get from high dose tablets however. Higher dose tablets should only be taken when deficiency has been diagnosed.

Like iron, your body accesses and regulates zinc best when you get it from animal foods so, again, vegetarians need to be more careful.

Selenium

Selenium is a powerful antioxidant that protects brain cells as well as bolstering the effects of some other antioxidant substances including vitamin C.

It's made health news in recent years with the discovery that people who have better selenium status have better brain health and the possibility that it also helps fight some cancers, especially prostate cancer.

If you are concerned that you might not be getting enough, get your doctor to check your selenium status but be very careful about taking large amounts in tablets. Like zinc and some other important minerals, selenium is toxic in very large doses (which you can only get from taking high dose tablets).

All minerals and most vitamins are best coming from food — the amounts foods contain are not excessively high and you get the benefit of the variety of other nutrients those foods also contain. There are lists in Chapter 4 of the foods supplying all the nutrients discussed here.

The antioxidant vitamins

Vitamin C
Vitamin C acts directly as an antioxidant, protects vitamin E and folate from degradation and is needed to make the substances that allow brain cells to communicate and function.

Science has shown that those who have low levels of vitamin C also frequently have lower cognitive abilities.

Vitamin E
Vitamin E is one of the most powerful nutritional antioxidants. It promotes efficient blood flow through the brain and elsewhere and plays an important role in the immune defense system.

Science has found that people with low levels of vitamin E have poorer memory and lower cognitive abilities but unfortunately taking it as a supplement doesn't seem to boost those abilities further, so the best plan remains eating food containing vitamin E.

What about nutrients or supplements to boost memory or brain function?

Unfortunately most pills and potions promoted as being able to boost your memory and save you from dementia fail to live up to their claims. You could spend quite a lot of money and they'd probably do little better than you could do by eating well and following the suggestions already given here.

Because we don't really know what causes dementia, it's hard to develop a medication that might prevent it but there is work underway all over the world trying to do that. So far, nothing does as well as exercise and a varied diet.

However, one multinational nutritional supplement company, in collaboration with medical and nutritional scientists, has developed a drink claimed to slow the progress of mild to moderate Alzheimer's disease. *Souvenaid*™ has been released in Australia accompanied by scientific research which suggests it might help. It contains a specific combination of many of the same nutrients and substances (mostly antioxidants) discussed in this chapter and in Chapter 4, though in a somewhat more concentrated form — DHA, EPA, choline, uridine, vitamin E, selenium, B12, B6 and folate originally from foods like seafood, meats, offal, eggs, dairy foods and vegetables and nuts. So should you rush out and buy this not inexpensive product? For those already facing cognitive decline or have early stage Alzheimer's, it certainly can't hurt to give it a try. Of course the bonus when you get these nutrients in natural foods, albeit in lower amounts, is that you also get protein and other nutrients as part of the bargain. But if you are struggling to eat enough food to get these important nutrients it is a concentrated alternative. Do your research and ask your doctor and dietitian.

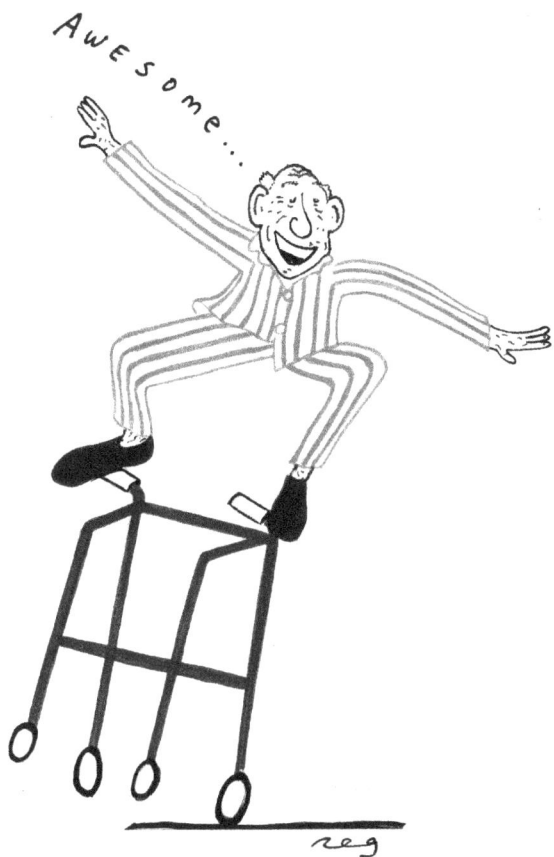

Awesome...

Chapter 3

EAT TO SHINE, EAT TO GLOW, EAT TO BEAT THE CREAKS

The blessings of a good appetite

Fabulous news! Yes, it's official: in older age you no longer need to accept a generous helping of guilt along with every mouthful of food. You have reached a milestone that signals you will probably be told to eat *more* rather than *less*, and that savoring every mouthful will be your secret to shining from now on.

There is more than one reason for this apparent turnaround and you've already heard about your body now needing more of some nutrients. From now on, allowing your appetite to trick you into eating too little is what you need to watch out for, as you will learn in Chapter 5, because weight loss poses a far greater risk to your health than do the few extra kilos you might be carrying.

Keeping your appetite sizzling so that you can keep eating well is one secret to 80 being the new 70.

I know that it will seem unthinkable to some readers that anyone could ever *not* feel like eating. But many of you will be able to attest that it certainly can and does happen.

But forewarned is forearmed: understanding what your appetite is up against as you get older gives you ammunition to counter its tricks and let you to shine on.

Lies and whispers — how and why your appetite deceives you

Appetite seems so simple: you eat when you're hungry and you don't when you're not.

But if it was that simple then why, when I look at food, especially if it's something delicious like a creamy dessert, do I get the message, 'hungry, hungry, hungry … must eat!' even though I know I don't *really* need it? And why are there also times when I have had a perfectly adequate meal, yet my appetite tells me I still *need* ice cream when any casual observer will realize that I just don't? I'm sure this is something many of you will easily identify with.

But the stark contrast is what I more often hear from my older clients, 'but I'm just not that hungry' or 'I'm full' after a few mouthfuls, when it really is obvious that three mouthfuls are not in any way an adequate meal. It's alarmingly common and if these messages are believed and too little food is eaten as a result, it's potentially very dangerous.

Your appetite is a response mechanism

For most of us, thankfully, food is not all about nutrition, but is also about our senses and about sharing and enjoying life. And that's the way it should be of course. You feel hungry when a whole barrage of signals combine — from habit, from our sense of taste, smell, sight, touch and even hearing, as well as from our stomachs and our intestines and from hormones and brain chemicals. The inconvenient truth is that changes can happen in any or all of these with age. Add the considerable effects of medications, illness and life events and all too soon you get those 'not hungry' messages and skip meals or eat less than you need.

Life events especially play a very big, often unrecognized part in your appetite. Everyone has had at least a couple of days of not feeling like eating when they were ill, but grief after the loss of someone close to you, or depression, or the stress of some sort of upheaval in your day-to-day life can also be appetite-killers.

As you advance in age it's dangerous to unquestioningly accept such messages as legitimate reasons not to eat. Your appetite helps feed you sufficiently to keep your muscles, bones and brain up to speed so the stakes are too high now to allow appetite mistakes to dictate how much you eat.

Your appetite may need a bit of TLC to get it back on track and that means accepting two important things:

1. You need to make a conscious effort to identify and then work around appetite mistakes

2. And from now on, even a small amount of *unintentional* weight loss shows that *you are not eating enough* no matter what your appetite may have been telling you.

I know it's difficult, if not nigh impossible to eat when your body is telling you that you're not hungry. In fact, for me, it's a lot harder than saying 'no' to chocolate chip icecream after dinner, but the stakes are too high to let the mistake take effect

Eating is habit forming, but so is *not* eating

When you were younger, even lengthy times of poor appetite were relatively insignificant because you could bounce back so easily. Once you are beyond 65 or so, any time your appetite is reduced for a few days, it's less likely to bounce back to what it was. Unless you work around that, you'll fall into the habit of eating less and that habit will become more and more embedded over the coming years.

What's the answer? Fortunately, it seems that eating itself is the cure, whether your appetite tells you to eat or not. The process of eating, especially when it happens frequently, in a mix of small meals, snacks and treats, can help bring your appetite back.

But I'm overweight. Surely not feeling like eating might mean losing some weight, and that's good, right?

No it's not; if weight loss happens only as a result of eating less, then it's more a hindrance than a blessing because you are risking your health and mobility, and therefore your independence.

As discussed in Chapters 1 and 5, the only way to reduce weight without also losing valuable muscle in your later age is by following a really good exercise plan suited to your health and mobility level, along with a well designed diet that includes plenty of protein.

The other big problem with a low appetite is that it's the all-important anti-aging protein foods like meats and fish, and meals with a good variety of colors that tend to get dropped first. If they get replaced, it's often by easier, comforting options like tea with a biscuit or toast, a piece of fruit, or smaller snacks low in nutrients so the protein is lost — as well as a raft of those other protectors of body and soul .

Forewarned is forearmed: understanding what influences your appetite

If your appetite is trying to thwart you, understanding what might be going on behind the scenes gives you the ammunition you need to counter its offensive. There can be lots of reasons:

1. Changes in your digestive system

As you eat, the appetite center in your brain receives messages from your stomach and the rest of the digestive system to give you that familiar feeling of fullness, and then reminds you in a few hours that it's time to eat again. This system unfortunately loses its accuracy as you get older so the wrong messages get relayed.

Age affects your digestive system in three ways:

- As food moves through your stomach and intestines, a number of hormones are also in action. They tell your body to slow your eating down so that food can be digested completely at each stage. As you age, changes in these hormones mean you get messages to slow eating down sooner than you should.

- The 'full' feeling that stops you eating is largely a result of signals from the stomach walls when they are stretched in specific ways by the food inside. But age changes the way your stomach walls stretch, causing those signals to be sent earlier than they should. As a result, you feel full before you really are, and stop eating sooner than you should.

- While you eat, and for some hours afterwards, food gradually moves out of your stomach into your intestine. It's when your stomach is nearly empty that messages are relayed to remind you it's time to eat again. But this process also often slows down considerably with age so, instead of being reminded it's time to eat your next meal after three or four hours, it can take much longer and you can feel like just one meal is able to keep you full most of the day.

Any, or all of these can be at play as you age, and all mean you are tricked into eating less than you really need.

2. Changes in your sense of taste and smell

As you age, you lose taste buds and your sense of smell diminishes. Both of these can also be further affected by illness and medications.

We all know how easy it is to eat entirely for the taste and smell of something delicious, and of course that's integral to the pleasure of food. So it's hardly surprising that you can lose enthusiasm for eating if these senses diminish.

What can help is finding ways to boost the appeal of your food, or sometimes choosing to eat just because you know you need it.

If your ability to taste has diminished so that food just doesn't have the appeal it once did, you may well find you need more salt, sugar or other flavor enhancers (herbs, sauces, gravies, cheese sauces, etc.) to stimulate your senses.

Too much salt or sugar can be unhealthy but, the older you become, it may be a matter of choosing the lesser of the evils for you. Eating too little and losing weight could pose a far greater risk to your health than the extra salt or sugar might.

If, at 85, a generous sprinkle of salt allows you to enjoy fish and chips, or if three spoons of brown sugar mean you eat a full bowl of porridge rather than two spoonfuls of porridge, then the benefits can easily outweigh the risks.

Interestingly, some types of food can boost taste better than others — unrelated to the amount of salt they contain — because they provide 'umami' or savory taste. This is a Japanese word meaning 'the essence of deliciousness' and it is our fifth sense of taste (along with sweet, sour, bitter and salty).

You need to determine what is right for you and discuss it with your doctor if necessary, but don't automatically accept that health messages aimed at younger people are appropriate for you when you are older; they are not.

3. Medications and how they play a part

It's an unfortunate fact that every medication, no matter how therapeutically effective, will often have at least one unwanted side effect. They may directly reduce your appetite by causing changes to the way food tastes — sometimes with an off-putting metallic taint — or drying out your mouth and making food less appealing and difficult to swallow, or causing nausea, diarrhea or constipation, with the result that your enthusiasm for eating is frequently a casualty.

But don't rush out and flush your medications into oblivion! These side effects don't affect everyone and, if they do, mostly wear off after a day or two. But it's worth being aware so you know the reason why your cheese on toast suddenly tastes like cardboard, or you inexplicably find yourself no longer enjoying your favorite ice cream. If these sorts of problems stick around any more than a day or so, a quick chat with your doctor can help sort them out. It might be possible to change the dosage or type of medication, or use something to tackle the symptoms while your illness is dealt with.

The problem is most likely to crop up when people take over-the-counter medicines, the ones you don't always think to discuss with your doctor. Common cold and flu tablets and liquids are very likely suspects, as are many combined preparations containing herbs, plant extracts, vitamins and the like, which are marketed to assist a huge variety of conditions including sleeping disorders, hair loss, anxiety and incontinence. We sometimes forget that any over-the-counter medication or alternative therapies, no matter how seemingly innocuous, have the potential for side effects by inter-reacting with medications we've been prescribed. It's always advisable to check with the pharmacist or with your doctor.

ENHANCING FLAVOR IN FOOD: UMAMI, GLUTAMATE AND MSG

All tastes are the result of food chemicals acting on our taste buds.

When table sugar, fructose from fruit or artificial sweeteners and other food components cause our taste receptors to react we taste it as 'sweet'.

We taste 'salt' when sodium chloride (table salt) or potassium chloride (sometimes marketed as 'no salt' brand) does the same to our salt receptors, and 'sour' as a result of a number of food components.

We also know that we taste umami flavor when glutamate (an amino acid from protein) and maybe other natural food chemicals cause our taste receptors to react.

The very interesting thing about umami flavor is that it also seems to be able to boost our appreciation of salty and sweet tastes so that we can get away with using less salt or sugar yet achieve the same taste.

Glutamate is found in many strongly flavored foods including cured meats (ham, salamis, etc.) marinated fish and strongly flavored fish like anchovies, dried and semi dried tomatoes, tomato paste, parmesan and other hard, strongly flavored cheeses, seaweed, mushrooms (especially dried), vegemite, soy sauce and Japanese miso.

There are also a number of food additives containing glutamate — MSG is one which is well known. Any manufactured food using dried cheese or powdered or dried tomato, hydrolyzed vegetable protein or soy sauce will be high in glutamates. These food additives are used to boost the taste of foods.

Years ago, MSG, in particular, was considered bad for you, and some people seem to react if they eat strongly flavored foods containing high levels of glutamate (including foods with MSG). But for the majority of people, who don't have a known glutamate intolerance, these concerns are overstated and may pale into insignificance when balanced against the dangers of eating too little food. If you are struggling to eat because foods lack taste, and you are not intolerant to glutamates, then they can do a lot to boost your enjoyment and help you eat better. And if you need to avoid high salt foods to reduce your sodium intake, MSG can help because you only need about a third as much as table salt to get a good savory flavor.

Interestingly too, glutamate stimulates saliva production so might even help if you suffer from a dry mouth.

There are a variety of things to keep in mind when it comes to medications and the greater the number you take, the greater chance one or a combination will have an effect.

- Even with something you have been taking for years, if a new medication is added to the mix it can bring on side effects you hadn't previously experienced.

- As you age, your body gets less and less efficient at getting rid of medications after they have done their job so their side effects can last longer, become more noticeable or become evident even though you may have been taking something for years with no problems.

- If you lose weight, you can end up needing less of many medications, so, unless the dosage is changed, side effects can start up or become more pronounced.

- Gastrointestinal upset (nausea, vomiting, diarrhea) is a very common problem with many medications, especially antibiotics, and of course it reduces your enthusiasm for food. Thankfully these sorts of issues are usually temporary. But because it's so important to keep eating its worth checking with your doctor whether there is anything you can do to reduce problems.

- Constipation also saps your appetite and is a side effect of many medications. For example, many common over-the-counter painkillers contain codeine, a cause of constipation. Of course vomiting and nausea for any reason will stop you eating so that needs to be dealt with as quickly as possible. (There are tips to counter nausea later in this chapter.)

- The number of prescription medications that can affect appetite is so extensive it's just not feasible to provide a comprehensive list here, particularly as problems often stem from the combined effect of two or more medications. The list here includes some of the most likely suspects, particularly those you can get without a prescription. But before you head to your doctor demanding change, first try employing strategies such as those listed later in this chapter in 'tips and tricks'. They can be enough to get you past temporary appetite and taste issues and return you to the habit of eating.

MEDICATIONS THAT MAY AFFECT APPETITE

This is by no means a complete list but many frequent categories include:

- Many blood pressure medications, particularly the ACE inhibitors
- Statins for lowering cholesterol
- Anti-reflux medications, particularly the PPIs
- Diuretics (fluid tablets)
- Anti-epileptic or antipsychotic medications
- Some antidepressants
- Antihistamines, mostly the older style but contained in many non-prescription cold and flu medications (including *Demazin, Mersyndol, Dimetapp*)
- The diabetes medication, metformin
- The opiates (including codeine) and NSAID (non steroidal anti inflammatory drugs) for pain relief.

4. Illnesses and medical procedures can affect appetite

Any time you are actively fighting illness or infection, it's normal for your appetite to decrease. But you now know how important food is in helping your body repair itself so you need to eat your way through illness now no matter what your appetite is telling you.

Your sense of taste and smell — essential to food enjoyment — can be affected if you have a cold, flu or an ear infection, if you have problems with your teeth, after a stroke or head injury, after surgery or radiation in your neck, head, ear or mouth. It's important to continue to eat if at all possible. Sometimes choosing different foods will help, sometimes swapping meals for high nutrition, high protein drinks for a while can get you through till your appetite returns. (See Chapter 8 for some suggestions.)

5. Nutrient deficiencies can affect appetite

Keeping your appetite firing is self-perpetuating because eating poorly (particularly if you have lost weight) means you can have easily missed out on vitamins and minerals including vitamin B1 (thiamine), magnesium, sodium, iron or zinc which can all cause a reduced appetite.

Zinc is especially important for your sense of taste, and deficiencies are common in older age.

If your appetite is down, blood tests to check for deficiencies should be a priority so any shortfall can quickly be rectified with food and supplements.

6. Stress, depression and grief affect appetite

As mentioned before, stress, including grief after losing a loved one, a serious illness or accident, anxiety over life events or depression, can cause a loss of appetite. Let's face it, in these circumstances eating can just seem so irrelevant. You may find your appetite completely absent for a while, or one mouthful will have you feeling full. You may also feel like your throat 'closes up' or your mouth feels too dry to swallow when you try to eat.

It's critical to be aware that eating is the path to preserving your independence and to thwarting the accelerated aging that can happen if you don't eat enough.

Depression in older people not only produces a low mood and emotional changes but often physical symptoms such as weight loss, insomnia and agitation. These physical symptoms mean depression often gets mistaken for other problems and, unfortunately, it's too often not diagnosed and therefore not treated as it should be. Depression is more than just short term stress. It's not a weakness but an illness that needs acknowledgment and treatment before its effects on your appetite send you on an increasingly downward health spiral.

Many strategies can help with depression: counselling, social involvement and medications all play a part. In fact, some medications used for depression can even boost appetite a bit, which is useful if you are also really struggling to eat.

Treat depression as the illness it is and discuss your options with your doctor.

7. Bowel issues affect appetite

Constipation causes reduced appetite. It makes sense when you think about it, although it is not widely recognized, even by doctors at times, but is a big factor in reduced appetite for very many people.

Lots of things can cause constipation including medications, digestive system problems and various illnesses or injuries, but it very often comes down to not eating a large enough quantity of food or something as simple as not drinking enough fluids, or not getting enough activity in your day.

Your bowels work better when you get a good quantity of food and fluids passing through them, and when the actions of muscles in your belly, hips, legs and even arms move your body whenever you are active.

One common cause of constipation is the codeine that's in many higher strength pain and cold medications. This, and other opioid medications (like morphine), can cause constipation. Be sure to discuss options with your doctor to avoid constipation. And if it's an issue for you, try to avoid taking over-the-counter medications containing codeine.

Have a look at Chapter 7 for more ways to keep your bowels moving.

Diarrhea, at the other end of the spectrum, also affects appetite. This can be an occasional problem causing only short-term issues but for many, particularly anyone suffering from IBS (Irritable Bowel Syndrome), it's much more than occasional and can reduce your appetite, or mean you choose to eat less to avoid the unpleasant consequences.

Because both chronic diarrhea and weight loss are so damaging, these problems need efficient medical management to reduce diarrhea quickly.

Nausea of course reduces appetite and food intake, and has many, many causes. Constipation can cause nausea, as can dehydration and many illnesses. But there are strategies you can use to reduce its impact.

If you have concerns that a medication you are taking might be contributing to your feeling nauseous, discuss it with your doctor; there may be alternatives open to you.

WHAT TO DO IF YOU ARE BATTLING NAUSEA

Nausea, whether caused by medications, illness or, ironically, by not eating will have you convinced that getting anything down is absolutely impossible. But in fact eating is often the way to deal with nausea.

In fact, not eating can be the culprit so you need to trick your body into getting enough to reverse this cause. The key is to take small amounts frequently and usually to start eating as soon as you wake. Just a sip or a small bite every 10 or 15 minutes is enough. And don't let up, because everything you can get is doing you good.

Sweet drinks (sweetened with normal sugar (sucrose) or glucose, NOT artificially sweetened) — from the fridge or with ice — are a good choice. You can get *Lucozade* (a commercial glucose soft drink) or for most people lemonade is fine — either straight or diluted, fizzy or allowed to go flat.

Ginger helps reduce nausea and can be taken in any form including ginger ale. Peppermint does the same so enjoy a cup of peppermint, ginger or regular tea, and add glucose powder or sugar to this also.

You can dilute these drinks if you need to with water if they taste too strong.

Many people find plain or slightly salty cracker biscuits good too, or a small handful of dry breakfast cereal. Nibble on these as soon as you get up, and about 10 or 15 minutes before meals to help you reduce nausea and get more out of your meals.

Ask your doctor about your medications. If any are contributing to your nausea, there may be alternatives you can take.

There are also special medications you can take before meals to help reduce nausea.

Ways to rekindle your love affair with food

So now that we've dealt with what causes appetite problems, here are a few things that might help you rekindle your appetite.

What to do if you are getting those *'not hungry'* messages:

First and foremost, watch your weight; if it falls, then you are not eating enough.

- Recognize the 'not hungry' messages as mistakes and try to eat anyway.

- Eat by the clock if you need to; have something every two to three hours. The mere act of eating, even in small amounts, can trigger a return of appetite if it's been slipping, as long as you keep it up. Missing meals will make matters worse.

- If you haven't yet lost weight but have been feeling less hungry, remember you still need to have at least three 'meals' *each* day to keep reminding your brain that it has an eating habit.

- If you have already lost weight, you need more 'meals' — 5 or 6 each day. You can have small amounts at each meal but each must contain high nutrition foods (such as in the lists at end of the chapter).

- If you just can't face your usual meals, take a commercial supplement or high protein drink between meals, or instead of meals if necessary (see suggestions in Chapter 8).

- Be kind to yourself, use treats to tempt your appetite between meals. You are allowed chocolate, cake, potato chips, lollies, icecream — go for whatever you *really* love. A few treats here and there along with more nutritious foods can remind your appetite that food is pleasurable *and* important.

Above all, don't give up, keep trying.

What to do if you feel full too soon and can't finish your meals?

Recognize that your capacity to eat can change but your stomach doesn't 'shrink' as old wives tales might have you believe. You cannot possibly be full on only two spoonfuls of food. Recognize the mistake.

Of course you don't want to eat till you feel ill, or make yourself sick by eating more than you really can take but there are a few tricks you can try:

- Have just one or two spoons more than you feel you want. They're little steps in triggering the return of your appetite.

- Have liquid meals — drinks or soups, etc. Liquids slip more easily through the stomach so can bypass the stomach's fullness sensors. (Choose from the options in Chapter 8 which are high in nutrition value.)

- Add lots of sauce or gravy to meals to make food more liquid.

- Split meals into two or three small portions and eat the whole meal over a few hours.

- If you are really struggling, have five to six small meals each day. This often makes getting enough food in easier.

- Make sure every mouthful you have is a nutritious one. If you can only get half a cup of food in at each meal, make sure it's packed with the most important nutrients for your body to regain health and independence.

Make sure you make the most of every small amount you can eat

I don't have to tell you that tea and toast will make you feel just as full as if you had added an egg or a slice of cheese to the toast, and you know how much more benefit you'll get from the added protein. It's always been that way, but it matters even more if you are eating less than you need.

A good tip is to eat the most nutrient-dense foods on your plate first. Choose protein foods first, then your colors: vegetables, fruits, and grain based foods. That way, you don't waste your precious appetite on foods that give you less nutrition. Once your appetite is back you can make amends.

The foods suggested in the Chapter 8 in Eating Plan 3 will help you boost the nutritional content in every mouthful you eat.

What can I do if my mouth feels dry or I feel like I can't swallow?

As you get older you produce less saliva and this can be exacerbated by medications that can make this condition even worse.

Saliva plays an essential role in your ability to taste foods, the health of your teeth and your ability to swallow smoothly. Without the lubrication of saliva, food may feel like its getting stuck or it becomes difficult to get out of your mouth and down to your stomach as easily as it once was.

If you are having difficulty swallowing and if you cough while you eat or drink, or straight after, it's important to have a chat with your doctor because that could mean small amounts of food or drink may accidentally be getting into your lungs instead of the esophagus. Even a few drops or a tiny crumb ending up where it shouldn't be can cause a chest infection.

The feeling that your throat closes up a bit as you eat can also be caused by stress and grief, and the strategies outlined below also apply in helping you continue to eat in these circumstances.

If you find getting food down is a struggle these strategies can help:

- Swap solid meals for nutritious drinks (see Chapter 8) or liquid meals such as soups or casseroles for a while.

- If problems crop up when you start a new medication then of course check with your doctor who may be able to give you something more palatable.

- There are also good products on the market to help lubricate your mouth.

- Make sure your meals have extra liquid in them or add extra sauces or gravy to your normal meals. Add cream, custard or ice cream to desserts.

- Stew your fruit or buy it canned in syrup or juice instead of fresh. The softer texture helps you to swallow.

- Have a drink on hand and sip it as you eat.

- Use flavor enhancers like salt, spices, sauces or even MSG or other glutamates in your food. You only need a very small amount to boost flavor and 'make your mouth water'.

The special value of treats — go on, it's okay to spoil yourself!

If your appetite is really challenged, 'treat' foods can really help. Even the thought of your favorite chocolate, a slurp of ice cream, a wedge of triple-cream brie, a nip of sherry, a doughnut, crispy fried fish, pork crackling, something from the patisserie, a perfect peach or couple of strawberries can get your mouth watering!

When you have absorbed a lifetime of nutrition negatives that nag at you to 'avoid eating this', 'don't have that', or 'cut down on these', you can end up thinking all the foods you love are bad for you. If your appetite is dwindling then changing to 'please have this' and 'enjoy that' and 'yes you can have these', can do wonders.

Once a day, or at least every couple of days, allow yourself a *real* treat — anything you used to really love. You don't have to eat it all, just a taste might do at first.

A small glass of wine, a sherry or a beer before or with a meal if you have been used to that can help your appetite too.

Treats may not contribute many nutrients, but if they help to re-ignite your appetite then they are worth it.

Spoil yourself, indulge yourself as long as you need. Very often you'll find your appetite returns. Remember the rules of eating have changed now you are older: **as long as you also eat the foods you need** there is absolutely no reason to worry about the 'don't haves' any more.

This is the time of your life when you are allowed those lovely treats. Remember, 'you're only old once' so enjoy them!

Chapter 4

NUTRIENTS TO HELP CHEAT AGING

This chapter is not going to discuss every nutrient people need — there are plenty of books that cover more general nutrition advice. Here, the focus is on those nutrients that have special or increased importance now you are older, that take into account extra wear and tear your body has encountered, inevitable changes in your digestive and other systems, illness history and the medications you take.

There is a bit of unavoidable overlap with some nutrients already discussed in Chapter 2 because of their special importance to the brain, but which also pop up here with wider implications for the rest of your body.

Before you read on, a reminder of what to consider when thinking about vitamin tablets or supplements:

Forget the idea that if small amounts of nutrients are recommended for good health, then large amounts must be even better, because it's just not true. Don't waste your money because you can really only use the vitamins and minerals immediately needed. Any extra amounts boost only the sewerage system, not your body. And excess intakes can set up imbalances between nutrients, interact with your medications and disrupt the smooth running of your body systems. Not only that, but Mother Nature gets the balance right when you source your vitamins and minerals from *a wide variety of foods*. Foods contain all sorts of other substances many of which work alongside nutrients to help us use them efficiently. When you replace food with tablets you forego any such benefits.

Supplements are of course invaluable if you are deficient, and there is unlikely to be harm in most general purpose multivitamin tablets supplying doses up to the recommended daily allowance. But it's important that you are sure you are deficient when you take any single vitamin and that your doctor knows about any you take if you haven't been tested for a deficiency.

Protein

You know already from Chapter 1 why protein and muscle are important, here is more information on how much you should get and why.

As you age, you may need as much protein as an elite athlete!

Amazing as it may seem, as your activity levels slow down with age, you body's need for protein can at times be close to that of an elite athlete. That's nearly double that of an average, less active adult.

Athletes need extra protein to keep their muscles up to scratch because of the extreme activity levels they subject themselves to. In older age, you may need extra protein because of the extra demands on your body through being unwell, surgery or illness, or compensating for any muscle losses. At these times you will probably need more than just food to get the protein required to help you recover, you may need to take a supplement.

Even without the stress of illness or muscle loss, and even if you feel and eat well, you have reached an age when you need to think of the amount of protein in each of your meals.

WHICH NUTRIENTS ARE ESPECIALLY IMPORTANT TO HELP YOU CHEAT THE RAVAGES OF AGE

Protein

Folate

Vitamin B12

Vitamin D

Vitamin K

The minerals:

    calcium

    magnesium

    iron

    iodine

The antioxidants:

    vitamins A, C and E

    minerals zinc and selenium

    phytochemical antioxidants

SERVES OF FOODS REQUIRED TO SUPPLY 10 GRAMS PROTEIN (APPROXIMATE)

Most people will need between 60 and 90 grams (2-3 ounces) of protein each day based on 1.2 grams (0.4 oz) for every kilogram you weigh, with more in times of illness and higher need.

Eggs	1 large egg
Cheese	1½ slices of cheese
	or 7 x 1 cm cubes cheese
	or 1½ tablespoons of cottage cheese
	or ⅛ small wheel of brie or other soft cheese
	or 2 cheese sticks
	or 2 tablespoons light cream cheese
Milk	1 cup of milk
	or ¼ cup milk powder
	or a small glass of a high protein supplement drink made using milk
Yoghurt	1 tub (150ml or 5oz) yoghurt — soy or dairy
Chicken	½ chicken thigh
	or 1 small drumstick
	or 2½ chicken nuggets
Fish	1 small piece of grilled fish (about matchbox size)
	or 2½ fish fingers
	or 6 medium prawns or oysters
	or ¼ cup (a bit less than a small can) of tuna or salmon
Lamb	1 small lamb chop or about a matchbox sized portion of other meat
	or 1 thick sausage
Bacon	1 rasher of bacon
	or 7 thin slices of salami
	or 1 slice of deli ham or other sliced meat

Pies	1½ party pies or sausage rolls
Bread	2 thick slices of wholemeal bread
	or 1½ slices soy and linseed bread
	or 3 toast slices white bread
Breakfast	2 cups of wholegrain breakfast cereal
	or 4 breakfast wheat biscuits
	or 1½ cups porridge
Pasta, rice	2 cups of pasta
	or 1 heaped cup of rice (cooked)
	or 1½ cups canned spaghetti in sauce
Beans	1 cup (about 200g) of baked beans
	1 cup of lentils or beans
Soy	100g of tofu (about the size of a pack of cards)
	or 1 cup (200ml or 6-7oz) soy milk
	or 1½ cups of soy-based high protein supplement
Nuts	40 to 50g of nuts (about ½ cup)
	For low volume, concentrated options check the lists of high protein drinks in Chapter 8 and commercial supplements in the appendix.

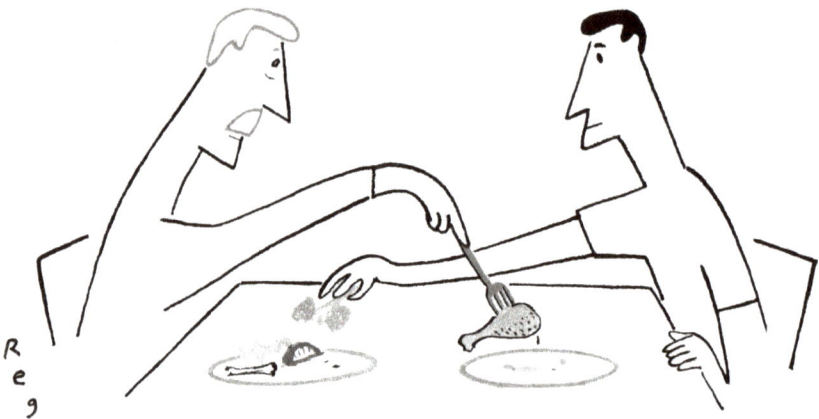

R
e
g

Getting enough of the right stuff

When you are well, getting the protein you need is usually as easy as building your meals around a good protein food and adding those multi-coloured vegetables, grains and fruits — at least at most meals. The exact amount each person needs depends on your weight and health so it's just not possible here to give an exact guide for each individual. Not only that, but while most experts agree that the amounts younger adults are advised to eat are too low, it will be a while before they all agree on exactly what to recommend for older folks.

For those who are mostly well, an amount of around 1.2 grams of protein for every kilogram you weigh (or 0.55g per pound weight) is often suggested as the ideal level (some researchers suggest 1.5 grams per kilogram per day – 0.68g per pound). That means 60 to 80g a day, spread as evenly as possible through the whole day, will usually be enough.

But there are lots of times when you are:

> recovering from illness,

> heading for surgery or have just had an operation

> immobilized (or have recently been) due to illness

> losing weight (and therefore muscle)

> exercising to boost your muscle

> moving into later old age

At these times you could need 15 or 20 grams *more* protein each day, the equivalent of *an extra*

> 2 small chops

> or 2 eggs

> or about 4 slices of wholemeal bread

> or 2 cups of cooked rice

> or 2 cups of lentils

If that sounds an impossible feat or you are struggling to eat enough, high protein drinks or a special supplement drinks (see Chapter 8) can make life easier.

Start to boost your protein intake as soon as you possibly can after illness or surgery to help your recovery — even if you are still laid up.

Don't always expect to be able to see improvements in the mirror but remember than an adequate protein intake will certainly help you regain strength and ability, as well as supporting your body in all those other important internal functions you've read about earlier in this book.

I don't eat meat — will I get enough protein?

If you have gradually cut down on animal protein foods but are not necessarily committed to vegetarian eating, you really need to reconsider your choices as you move into your older age. As you've heard already, it's generally much easier to get enough protein from animal foods because you can get what you need from smaller amounts of food, not to mention the easy-to-access iron, zinc, selenium and vitamin B12 they supply.

If you have cut out meat but still eat dairy foods and eggs then you may need to take iron and maybe other supplements, but you shouldn't have problems getting the protein you need.

But if you have chosen to be vegetarian, then you need to be extra vigilant about the protein you eat, as well as the nutrients you need. Nuts, pulses (lentils and beans), seeds, grains and soy products such as tofu are all good options. You can also take high protein supplements made from soy, rice or other plant proteins like pea protein.

Getting enough folate

Folate (also in foods as folic acid) is a B vitamin essential for peak brain function. It also protects against bowel cancer (and possibly other types) and helps keep blood levels of homocysteine down. You can read more about homocysteine in the box in this chapter but what is important to know is that this is a substance which, when allowed to accumulate in the bloodstream, is associated with heart disease and Alzheimer's dementia.

Folate is found in quite a variety of foods (and is now added to many commercial breakfast cereals and some fruit juices) so most people will be able to avoid a deficiency but there are many medications that either affect how well folate is absorbed from your food, or change the way it's used in the body and if you have been taking any of these medications for a while, your folate status should be regularly checked with a blood test.

A mild deficiency of folate might set you on a path to heart or cognition problems. A severe deficiency can cause diarrhea, loss of appetite, weight loss, weakness, sore tongue, headaches, heart palpitations, irritability and forgetfulness.

The common NSAID (non steroidal anti inflammatory drug) pain relievers on the list of medications here, including ibuprophen and aspirin, are worth a special mention (not paracetamol — *Panadol* — which is a different type of pain relief medication). Because you can buy them at a supermarket or chemist without a prescription so many people believe them to be completely safe and may take them often enough to affect folate levels. If you do take them regularly without a script, let your doctor know. You may need to try alternative medications or take folate supplements if there is an issue. Other NSAIDs cause similar problems but are only available on prescription, and your doctor can easily monitor them.

Very low dose aspirin such as *Cartia* 100, *Cardiprin* 100 brands are often prescribed to help reduce the 'stickiness' in the blood and thus avoid heart attack and stroke. These low dose tablets don't cause the problems higher doses of most NSAIDs do, but your folate status should be monitored regularly if you take them routinely.

You get folate from green vegetables, especially the leafy ones like kale and spinach, but also broccoli, as well as liver, commercial breakfast cereals and juices with added folate, nuts, chick peas, and yeast or vegetable extracts such as *Vegemite* and *Marmite*. Folate is also included in the complete nutrition food supplement drinks listed in the appendix and Chapter 8.

Before you think of taking folate as a tablet, a word of caution: get a test to check if you are deficient first because getting too much folate on its own can also be harmful. Usually a blood test for folate will also check your vitamin B12 levels because these two vitamins are dependent on each other.

And be extra careful if you have reduced kidney function. Taking high doses of folate alone or in very high doses with other B vitamins in tablet form can worsen any kidney damage. While most lower dose combined-B vitamin supplements contain both folate and B12 in amounts that won't cause you harm, you must always discuss taking any vitamin or mineral supplement tablet with your doctor to avoid causing yourself extra problems.

MEDICATIONS THAT MAY AFFECT FOLATE STATUS

(brand names are in italics and may vary depending on the country of purchase)

Metformin for diabetes	including *Diabex, Diaformin, Formet, Glucobet, Glucophage, Glucophage XR, Metex*
Sulphasalazine used in IBS, Crohn's disease and ulcerative colitis	including *Salazopyrin, Salazopyrin SR, Pyralin EN*
Phenytoin anticonvulsant/anti epileptic	*Dilantin*
Methotrexate used in cancer therapy and rheumatoid arthritis	*Methoblastin*
Triamterene, a diuretic	*including Hydrene 25/50*
Barbiturates (sedatives, not often used nowadays)	other names amylobarbitone and amobarbital
Some blood lipid lowering fibrates	including fenofibrate (*Lipidil*)
Non-steroidal anti-inflammatory medications (NSAIDs) for mild or moderate pain, fever and inflammation relief	Available without prescription — including ibuprofen: (*Nurofen, Advil* and generics) naproxen (*Naprosyn*), and aspirin
	Others available only on prescription include:
	diclofenac (*Voltaren*), celecoxib (*Celebrex*), meloxicam (*Mobic*), piroxicam (*Feldene*), indomethacin (*Indocid*), mefanamic acid (*Ponstan*), ketoprofen (*Orudis*)

A NOTE ON HOMOCYSTEINE

If you read up on health topics you may have heard mention of homocysteine and how it's bad for your heart and might cause stroke and Alzheimer's disease, and that is certainly true if the levels in your blood are too high.

But homocysteine in just the right amount has an important role to play too. It comes from the proteins we eat and, with the help of the vitamins folate, B6 and B12, is used to make two substances that are very good for you, one of which is a powerful antioxidant called glutathione.

Homocysteine is only a problem when it builds up in your blood because it doesn't get converted into glutathione, which happens if your levels of these B vitamins are too low. Keeping homocysteine levels just right depends on making sure you don't become deficient, but unfortunately taking extra vitamins beyond that doesn't add extra benefit. You might hear some big claims made that various supplements reduce homocysteine levels, but always check with your doctor before taking these vitamins in tablet form. Taking them when you are not deficient can cause you harm.

You might also hear about supplements of glutathione itself with claims that it will help but, sadly, the reality is that these don't get absorbed well enough to be of much use, despite their considerable cost, so will probably give you little or no benefit.

Vitamin B12

Vitamin B12 deficiency is worryingly common in older age, and because it shares some symptoms with dementia it's of particular concern, as you've already heard. B12 is essential for correct functioning of nerves and for making healthy blood cells, and a deficiency can cause confusion, difficulty concentrating, memory loss, irritability, depression, anemia, fatigue, shortness of breath, tingling and numbness in the limbs, loss of balance and reduced appetite. It also works with folate in homocysteine conversion, so a deficiency can cause higher levels of homocysteine in the blood.

We get B12 almost exclusively from animal foods, so vegetarians — in older age especially — should always take a B12 supplement for this reason. But, as with all nutrients and particularly this one, getting enough depends equally on how well we can absorb it from our food as it does on eating food containing B12.

B12 deficiency gets more common as you get older mainly because of age-related changes in your stomach and intestines that make you less able to absorb this vitamin. It needs just the right amount of acid from your stomach to help absorption and two things affect those levels: firstly, you make less acid as you get older and secondly, medication for reflux reduces acid production further — and both lessen absorption. As well, you can miss out on B12 if you suffer recurrent gastrointestinal upset or diarrhea as you may in IBS, or as a side effect of antibiotics, or due to other illness.

And finally, possibly the biggest contributor, if you gradually cut down on eating meat and other animal foods as you get older you set yourself up for a B12 deficiency.

If any of these issues apply to you, or if you take medications listed here, you must have your B12 levels checked regularly.

LIST OF COMMON ANTI-REFLUX MEDICATIONS WHICH MAY AFFECT B12 LEVELS WHEN USED OVER A NUMBER OF YEARS

(Brand names are shown in italics and may vary depending on the country of purchase)

The PPIs (proton pump inhibitors):	Esomeprazole (*Nexium*)
	Lansoprazole (*Zoton*)
	Omeprazole (*Losec, Prohibitor*)
	Pantoprazole (*Somac*)
	Rabprazole (*Parief*)
The H2 blockers are less likely to cause problems but also reduce stomach acid so having B12 status checked is prudent in late age.	Ranitidine (*Zantac, Rani, Ranitidine*)
	Cimetidine (*Tagamet*)
	Nizatidine (*Tazac*)
	Famotidine (*Amfamox, Pepcidine*)

Vitamin D

A vitamin D deficiency is a big problem affecting up to one third of people in Australia and is more likely in older age. In aged care facilities, that figure jumps to over half of the residents!

Most people will know vitamin D is essential for bones, but it's far, far more than that. Insufficient vitamin D also causes weakness and pain in your large muscles, affecting walking. It is thought to contribute to heart disease, certain cancers (colorectal, breast and prostate particularly), depression and diabetes and some other illnesses. In fact, if your levels are low when you are older you have a higher chance of succumbing to illnesses and even dying from a number of causes.

Unlike most vitamins, you only get small amounts of vitamin D from foods naturally. Most of what you need, you produce yourself through your skin when you are in the sun. In our modern lives, now that we don't get the same sun exposure our forebears did, we risk not getting enough vitamin D.

VITAMIN D DEFICIENCY

A vitamin D deficiency can cause:

Weakened bones, increasing your chance of a fracture if you fall

Weakness and pain in large muscles, particularly those of your thighs and buttocks increasing your chances of falling

Hypertension (high blood pressure) and cardiovascular problems.

Deficiency may also contribute to:

An increased risk of colorectal and other cancers

Your chance of developing diabetes

An impaired immune response to infectious illnesses

Depression and anxiety.

If you tend to be involved in mostly indoor activities, work indoors, find it difficult to get outside, or if you choose to avoid the sun for other reasons such as skin cancer concerns, then you are very likely not getting enough vitamin D. If you are out and about every day, gardening, fishing, walking or doing other similar outdoor activities and exposing at least your arms and some of your legs and face without sunscreen for about half an hour most days, then you might be able to get what you need. But for anyone else, and during winter especially, choosing foods with vitamin D and adding supplements to make up any shortfall is the way to go.

If you are not sure, ask your doctor to arrange a blood test to have your vitamin D status assessed. If your levels are just a bit low, or if they are fine *but* you are not getting any sun, a low dose supplement each day is probably needed. If you are found to be deficient you may need a higher dose, and it can take a few months to get those levels back up.

FOOD SOURCES OF VITAMIN D

The effect of sunlight on the skin is the body's best source of vitamin D, but some foods do contribute:

Fish liver oil (e.g. cod liver oil)

Oily fish (salmon, sardines, herrings, mackerel)

Butter, and margarine with added vitamin D

Small amounts in meat, milk and eggs

Field mushrooms grown outdoors and naturally exposed to the sun before harvesting

Commercial mushrooms specifically exposed to UV radiation before packing to boost vitamin D (indicated on packaging).

Unless you eat a lot of the foods listed above and if you don't regularly go out in the sun, then a supplement is generally advisable.

Vitamin K (and warfarin)

Vitamin K is needed to clot your blood to stop you bleeding when your skin is damaged. It's an essential vitamin and is found in green vegetables, wheat germ and the foods listed here. But some medical conditions can cause blood to clot inside your blood vessels when it shouldn't. This can cause stroke and heart attack. To avoid this, or if you have already suffered such an event, you may be prescribed the drug warfarin (brand names include *Coumadin, Marevan in Australia*).

Warfarin works by acting against vitamin K in the body. The amount of warfarin you take is balanced against your vitamin K intake to get your rate of blood clotting just right for your condition (the degree of clotting is assessed by the INR blood test which is done regularly once you are on warfarin).

Many, many people who take warfarin believe they must stop eating foods with vitamin K completely to get their INR right, but it is a balance that's needed. The foods that contain vitamin K also supply lots of other essential nutrients (like folate, vitamin C and many different antioxidants) so cutting them out is just not a good idea.

What you need to do instead is plan to eat about the same amount of food containing vitamin K each day and then your dose of warfarin gets balanced against that. Check the list here and vary the types of foods you choose from the list as much as you like as long as you have around the same amount of vitamin K each day.

BALANCING FOOD SOURCES OF VITAMIN K

The following quantities of foods provide about the same amount of vitamin K:

Asian greens, all varieties: ½ cup cooked

Asparagus: 8 medium spears

Beetroot leaves — NOT the beetroot itself: ½ cup

Broccoli: ½ cup cooked

Cabbage (darker green/red varieties): 1 cup

Endive: 1 cup

Herbs — basil, coriander, rocket, parsley (fresh, green herbs): approx ½ cup in total should be counted, but amounts less than that, included as part of a recipe for more than just one person, or used as garnish, pose no problem

Kale: ½ cup cooked

Lettuce — 'fancy', darker types: 1 cup

Spinach/silverbeet: ½ cup cooked

Mix these foods up as you wish, just make sure you get approximately the same amount of vitamin K-containing food each day. To maintain variety, perhaps have a mix of broccoli and kale one day, spinach another, mix coleslaw with four spears of asparagus another, and a stir-fry with Asian greens on another day.

It shouldn't really affect your INR at all if you are only having a sprinkle or a teaspoon of herbs (or even if you use half a cup in a dish for a few people), one or two asparagus spears, a few bits of broccoli in a stir fry or a scattering of dark green or red lettuce in a salad mix.

There are also herbal preparations and supplements which, although they don't contain vitamin K, can affect your INR in other ways. If you are considering taking any of these, discuss it first with your doctor or dietitian:

Chamomile (in large amounts, not an occasional cup of tea)

Cranberry juice (more than one glass a day)

Omega-3 supplements (such as fish oil)

Garlic capsules (i.e. high dose garlic, not what you have in meals unless you eat a number of whole cloves at once)

Ginko biloba, ginseng, fenugreek tablets

Green tea in large amounts

Iron, magnesium or zinc supplements (usually okay if taken two hours before or after warfarin)

Glucosamine, chondroitin (usually taken for joint pain)

Vitamin E in large doses.

Calcium

You probably know that calcium is needed for strong bones, but it also helps your muscles work properly and plays an extremely important part in sending the messages that keep your heart contracting properly.

For most people, dairy foods (or soy and other milks with added calcium) are by far the most important sources, but calcium also comes from fish with edible bones (such as canned salmon or sardines), as well as from sesame seeds and some nuts (almonds, brazil nuts, hazelnuts), dried figs and broccoli. If these non-animal foods are your only source of calcium, you usually need to eat larger amounts to be sure to get enough calcium.

To get calcium from food, however, you also need vitamin D to absorb and use it properly. You may also lose calcium if you eat too much salt because that can cause the kidneys to get rid of calcium unnecessarily.

Ideally, some dairy food at each meal, plus at least one extra calcium food per day should be adequate for most people.

If you do take calcium supplements, don't take huge amounts because they are less well absorbed, and choose one that includes vitamin D to help absorption.

Magnesium

Magnesium is a remarkable nutrient, active in a huge number of body processes. It's important in coordinating muscle contraction, nerve transmission, maintaining the rhythm of your heart, producing healthy bone, releasing energy from food, building protein for muscle tissue and assisting with blood glucose control.

We get magnesium from nuts and nut butters, whole grains (but it's lacking in white and more refined grain foods), brown rice, soy beans and soy products like tofu, green and leafy vegetables, dried fruits and sundried tomatoes and fish.

As you get older, your ability to absorb magnesium from food diminishes, and any gastrointestinal upset makes that worse. Some medications also affect magnesium absorption, including the fluid tablets lasix (*Frusemide*) and hydrochlorthiazide (*Microzide*), and some antibiotics (e.g. gentamicin, amphotericin). Combine this with eating less food, and a magnesium deficiency can occur.

Iron

Iron deficiency unfortunately becomes quite common as people age and is a very debilitating condition. It causes anemia and, as a result, fatigue, sleeplessness, headaches, poor appetite and nausea. Some physical signs include 'spoon' nails (where your fingernails have a spoon shape), a sore mouth and a tendency to look pale.

You have also read earlier that a milder form of iron deficiency causes cognitive decline and that stands to reason because iron helps transport and store the oxygen needed for every activity of every one of your cells, and the brain's needs are so much higher than anywhere else in the body. It's important to keep an eye on this because the longer an iron deficiency continues — even a mild one — the less likely any decline in brain or nerve function can be turned around by treatment.

If you are a red meat eater then your chances of having an iron deficiency are usually low: red meat is by far our most concentrated and most easily absorbed source of iron (especially the offal meats like heart, kidney and liver — lambs fry). Other meats and fish are also good sources, but if you don't eat much meat then you need to take extra care to get enough iron.

Like many other nutrients, iron is not easy to absorb from foods and as you get older this becomes more and more apparent. You also lose iron from your body if you bleed. As you get older, even small amounts lost over time from your stomach lining and intestines due to ulcers or inflammation — and combined with more frequent damage from increasingly fragile skin — can be enough to tip the balance.

Iron, like vitamin B12, needs stomach acid for efficient absorption and you have read how that declines with age and medications. Surprisingly, some food and drinks make it more difficult to get iron from your meals. Tea is one, so, as you get older, it's very important to avoid drinking tea with your meals. Leave at least and hour between eating a meal and having your cup of tea (that doesn't apply to green tea, herbal tea, infusions or coffee).

Fortunately, foods containing vitamin C — citrus fruits and many vegetables — boost your absorption of iron. A glass of orange juice helps you absorb iron from breakfast cereal, and a mix of vegetables helps you get iron from the meat and vegetables that have iron.

If your levels are low, you may be prescribed iron tablets. Unfortunately some people find the tablets difficult to tolerate and they can cause nausea, abdominal pain and constipation. Most people can, of course, avoid any of these problems by eating high iron-containing foods at least at two meals a day. But if you do need to take tablets, then splitting your iron dose over the day can help. Taking the tablets with a vitamin C food such as fruit juice at same time also helps. But certainly don't take your iron tablets with, or close to drinking your cup of tea.

Iodine

Iodine is vital for your thyroid function and is important for your brain health and keeping your body processes regulated. The amount of iodine that foods contain depends on how much is in the soil, and in Australia, unfortunately, those levels are low. Years ago iodine was commonly added to table salt to boost the amount people ate but now people often avoid salt or eat 'gourmet' salt (sea salt crystals, pink salt, etc.) which don't contain iodine. We also used to get a lot from milk and dairy foods but that came from iodine-based cleaning products used in dairies, a practice which is now out of favor, so dairy foods don't supply the iodine anymore they once did.

It's likely many older people don't get enough iodine.

Iodine is found in high levels in seaweed, so eaters of Japanese foods like sushi do well, but you also get it from most seafood, especially shellfish, and of course from foods prepared with iodine-containing salt.

The Antioxidants

Vitamin A (beta carotene and retinol), vitamin C, vitamin E, selenium, zinc and phytochemicals

You already know how important antioxidants are, and they gain elevated status the older you get as the tiny bits of damage done by free radicals accumulate over the years. That damage is not only in your brain of course, it's in every cell, in every organ. Unfortunately the jury is out on whether they are able to reverse any damage already done, but one great thing is that, as long as food is your source of antioxidants, you really can't get too much and every bit extra you do get will be of value.

As you read in Chapter 2, there are all sorts of other nutritional substances in the same foods that are also beneficial. Recent research has found that two antioxidant substances, lutein and zeaxanthin (and its associated xanthans), are especially important for your eyes in helping avoid damage that can lead to cataracts and macular degeneration. These substances are found in dark green vegetables like kale, broccoli and spinach and the yellow pigments in many foods including eggs.

Tea (white, green or the more familiar black) is also a great source of a number of antioxidants but it's best drunk between meals as drinking tea with your meal can reduce your absorption of some other important nutrients, especially iron. Herbal teas and infusions generally contain fewer antioxidant substances and don't cause problems with iron absorption.

ANTIOXIDANTS IN FOOD

There are hundreds of different kinds of antioxidants and related substances in foods, many of which also contribute to the colour of foods. You may have seen the term 'phytochemicals' which means chemicals in plants because most antioxidants come from plant foods, but they are also in some animal foods. Many foods contain a mix of different types of antioxidant so they appear more than once in this table.

Antioxidant	Source
The carotenoids	
lycopene, carotene	In citrus fruits (including marmalade because quantities are high in skin and pith), yellow and orange fruits and vegetables, apples, tea, tomatoes and all tomato products, watermelon.
lutein, zeaxanthan	In kale, spinach and similar leafy green vegies, sweet corn, yellow and orange vegetables and fruit, egg yolks, pink-fleshed fish and seafood (including salmon and prawns).
The polyphenols	
flavanoids	In darker green vegetables like kale and spinach, broccoli, parsley, black teas, coffee (but not instant coffee) seaweed and all sorts of soy foods (isoflavanoids).
anthocyanins	In red and purple fruits and vegetables including berries, red grapes and red wine, plums, eggplant skin, cherries, red lettuce or other vegetables with red or purple colour, raw cocoa powder and dark chocolate.
catechins	In apples, cocoa, white and green tea.
curcumin (turmeric spice)	This is the dark yellow spice used commonly in many Indian, Asian and middle eastern dishes.
other polyphenols	In coffee, green and black tea, whole grains, onions, garlic, ginger, mushrooms, flax seed, sesame seeds, lentils.

uridine	In tomatoes, brewer's yeast, broccoli, liver, molasses and nuts.
choline	In egg yolk, meats and fish, whole grains.
vitamin A	In all yellow and orange vegetables and fruits as well as in eggs, butter, milk, cheese and liver.
vitamin C	In citrus fruits, berries, mango, capsicums, potatoes, cabbage, spinach and Asian greens.
vitamin E	In wheatgerm (in wholemeal and wholegrain bread and cereals), vegetable oils, nuts, eggs, seeds, fish and avocado.
selenium	In nuts (especially brazil nuts) fish, seafood, liver, kidney, red meat, chicken, eggs, mushrooms and grains. (The level of selenium in foods usually depends on how much is in the soil in which the food is grown.)
zinc	In lean red meat, liver, kidney, chicken, seafood (especially oysters), milk, whole grains, legumes and nuts.

Vitamin A (including beta carotene and retinol)

Vitamin A is needed for good eyesight, to help you resist infection and keep your skin healthy. It also plays a role in cancer prevention and its antioxidant capabilities and the known benefits for your skin make it one you might read about for its 'anti-aging' abilities. If you are tempted to take large amounts you should know that too much vitamin A, taken as a supplement (particularly as retinol above 3000 micrograms or 10,000 IU per day) may cause liver damage and even increase your risk of hip fracture when you age.

Even when you are eating small amounts of food, it's rare not to get enough vitamin A. It's only when your intake has been very low for a while that a deficiency is likely, and then you will probably be low in many more nutrients than just vitamin A.

This is definitely one you need to check with your doctor before taking in a supplement.

Vitamin C

Vitamin C is essential in healing wounds, in keeping your teeth, gums and bones healthy. As well as being an important antioxidant, vitamin C also helps you fight infection and assists in getting iron from food.

It's commonly claimed to be useful for all sorts of problems and at much higher doses than you could ever eat in food. It has even been touted as an anti-aging substance but unfortunately there isn't much science to back up those claims. Most foods containing vitamin C are also great sources of all sorts of other antioxidants so you'll get the best benefits if you get this vitamin from foods.

Vitamin E

It's the powerful antioxidant role vitamin E plays that makes it so important in aging, but it's also vital for maintaining the health of each body cell and plays a central role in protecting you from cancer and heart problems. It just doesn't seem to give the same benefits when taken in tablet form as it does when sourced in foods so, like most nutrients, eating foods containing vitamin E remains the most beneficial.

Selenium

The importance of selenium to your brain and cognition has been discussed in Chapter 2. Its major role is as an antioxidant and, apart from its function in brain health, it also regulates your immune system, protects some other antioxidants including vitamin C, and is important for your thyroid function. It's also been touted as protecting against cancer of the prostate and other types of cancers, which has led to some people taking high doses. In excess, it's unfortunately quite toxic and there is nothing that proves levels higher than the recommended daily intake are needed; it's only selenium *deficiency* that sets up problems.

The amount of selenium in many foods depends on its levels in the soil and levels are low in Australia so getting enough can be a challenge. You probably need to eat brazil nuts, seafood, eggs or meat at least twice a day, or a supplement may be worth discussing with your doctor (either a general multivitamin or a commercial supplement drink will contain selenium).

Zinc

Zinc is essential for healing wounds, fighting infection, your sense of taste and your appetite. It's also recently been found that zinc, taken with the antioxidants vitamin C, vitamin E and beta-carotene may help you avoid macular degeneration. Unfortunately, taking extra if you are already getting enough doesn't boost any of these but being deficient is certainly a problem, especially once you are older.

Even a mild deficiency will make you more susceptible to infection and have you struggling to repair wounds.

A deficiency can also change the way food tastes and reduce your appetite — big issues to be avoided if you want to continue to eat well.

Zinc is more easily gained from animal foods (oysters are highest, also red meats, chicken, fish and seafood) and eating less of these foods over the years is often the main contributor to a zinc deficiency. The plant sources of zinc unfortunately also often contain a type of fibre that holds onto the zinc so it gets passed out in your feces instead of being absorbed into the blood. If you rely on plant sources of zinc you'll need to have your blood levels checked regularly to avoid problems.

Chapter 5

CAN YOU REALLY BE TOO RICH? TOO PAMPERED? TOO FAT? TOO THIN?

What *should* you weigh?

Here's where *being older* is suddenly the *best* thing. The quick answer at least to the boring old question about what you should weigh is: 'whatever you weigh now, don't go losing any!'

Not having to lose weight might not be the impression you get from the latest diets in glossy magazines, from what's being blasted at you by your TV, on the web, or even from the advice of some doctors, dietitians and self appointed health gurus. But that's pretty much because all that advice is for those youngsters out there. It might be great advice for the 30, 40 or 50-year-olds but you have finally escaped the endless 'diet to lose weight NOW' mantra.

The science is clear: weight loss diets, once you are in your late 60s or beyond, are *not* good news.

Losing weight by dieting from now on — no matter how good the diet sounds — means losing muscle and while that might not be obvious, either in your everyday activities or in how you look, we now know that it sets you up for ill health and squandering your independence.

Sure, if you lose weight, some of that might be fat, but since muscle will always have gone along with that, it's not a plus in the end: maybe it's not possible to be too rich (as Wallis Simpson once famously said), but it is certainly possible to be too thin.

There *is* a way to lose weight without losing muscle

The answer is *exercise*, not diet.

Even if 60 is the new 50, and 70 the new 60, you need to keep moving. Your muscles need to be reminded of their essential role by your staying active and teaching them new skills. You need to support them by eating as the previous chapters have been espousing, and then your muscles will still be there for you when you need them.

It might take a magic mirror to reflect the Venus or Adonis you know is inside you somewhere when your gym body seems to be have been mysteriously replaced by a wax replica that looks as if it has been left out in the sun, but every bit of muscle in your body is adding life to your years.

Unfortunately, I more often see older people who have lost four or five kilos (8 or10 lbs) without any conscious effort at all, and that's not good news. The muscle reduction as a result of that weight loss can already be affecting your health without you even being aware of it.

I know that for those of you who have always being a bit fatter than you 'should be' and struggled for years to keep your weight down, this is a mix of bitter and sweet: bitter because if you find you've lost weight you are going to feel virtuous, even smug, but along comes an annoying dietitian now saying *you shouldn't have!* But it's also sweet because finally it's okay to not be 'on a diet'.

But surely obesity is bad for your health?

Yes it is bad. Obesity in younger age sets you up for all sorts of health issues. In fact the grim truth is that too many people who have been obese throughout their lives don't actually make it into their 80s. But the time to lose excess weight is well before your late 60s. From now on, if you are very overweight it's really too late to do it safely *by yourself.*

If the excess kilos or pounds you carry have brought on or are worsening your diabetes, if they make getting around harder, or worsen joint, arthritic or other issues, then carrying less weight would of course make life easier and reduce your chances of further health problems. But trying to do anything about your weight *only by dieting* will do more harm than good; you must also exercise to head off muscle loss. Any exercise you can do yourself is great but a thorough medical examination before you begin anything new is highly advisable.

The exercises outlined in Chapter 1 to maintain and boost muscle will give you a guide, but you are best with a structured program designed specifically for what you need and what you are able to do, *and* you must commit yourself to continuing with it from now on.

But there's also the effect of inactivity on your health. In fact that's what more often drives obesity: the time you spend sitting, lying down and generally relaxing over the years. It may be good for the soul, and some down-time is important in your day-to-day life, but the balance has been thrown out of kilter by modern life. We just have far too much inactive time available to us and have become far too used to enjoying it. Every minute you are inactive reduces the time you are up and about burning kilojoules and boosting muscle. No matter what you weigh, if you spend less time watching TV, sitting at the computer or in an armchair, driving in the car or sitting on a bus and more time just being up and about, moving around will help your body and your brain, even if it doesn't strip off any kilos.

Ruth's story

Ruth had been a large lady since having her children. She was not an active person and had suffered a number of health and mobility problems since her late 50s.

She moved into a hostel in her late 60s when she needed a bit more help and wasn't able to get on the bus as well as she had.

By her late 70s, her mobility was quite reduced and the nursing supervisor in the hostel suggested she should see a dietitian to help her lose weight.

I was asked to see Ruth.

She was a lovely, friendly lady and, on the BMI chart, was certainly in the weight category of very overweight-to-obese. She had good friends in the hostel and they did all the bus trips and went out for coffee at least two or three times a week even though she was wheelchair-bound most of the day. She kept a supply of sweets and other treats in her room 'for the grandkids' and to 'share with the nurses'.

Ruth's diet was, in fact, quite good. She was not eating extreme amounts of kilojoules and had not gained any weight for years. Certainly Ruth would have been better able to get around if she was lighter and it was understandable that the nurses thought it a good idea for her to lose weight. But she wasn't able to do the exercise needed to maintain her muscle through weight loss. Changing her diet so she lost weight would have been harmful to Ruth and put her at higher risk of illness, not to mention restricting some foods that brought joy to her life.

Fortunately the hostel had access to a physiotherapist so we were able to discuss possible exercise options for Ruth and she was able to start on some very gentle workouts. But they really weren't enough to achieve much muscle building, if any.

Here was a lady who, at nearly 80, enjoyed her meals, and whose main source of pleasure in life revolved around the treats she shared with her grandchildren and her friends at their coffee sessions. Looking at the bigger picture, it just was not going to be possible to get Ruth to lose weight without harming her health and severely impacting the enjoyment she gained from life.

The advice to the facility had to be that weigh loss was not advisable for Ruth at her age.

It was a very different picture though for Margaret.

Margaret's story

Again, Margaret was a lady in her late 70s who was very overweight, had been for years and was starting to struggle in getting around as well as she would have liked. She had been diagnosed with type 2 diabetes only in the last year and was taking medication for high blood pressure.

Margaret was advised to attend a local gym program especially designed for seniors and started on a program of exercises and activities to strengthen her muscles and increase her exercise capacity. While she found it very hard at first, the boost to her energy levels and improvement in her ability to do everything from carrying the shopping to pushing her grandkids in the stroller made it worth the effort, and after a short while she began to really enjoy her sessions. She even felt she was enjoying the rest of life more and, much to her relief, was able to reduce her blood pressure medication and even avoid having to take medication for her diabetes at all.

Her diet wasn't restricted as part of her training, but she was assisted by the dietitian to plan meals and snacks with plenty of different foods, making sure she got the protein she needed. The treats she was so fond of were not forbidden, but she did find she was eating fewer of them as she varied her meals more and felt better.

Her weight didn't change much but she was stronger, healthier and felt far happier.

Exercise is not completely out of reach, no matter how overweight or how frail you may be. What is important is planning activities that are medically and physically appropriate.

What about the link between being overweight and type 2 diabetes — shouldn't I be worried?

Type 2 diabetes is a major health issue but, in older age especially, *lack of exercise* plays a bigger role than being significantly overweight. When muscle is active it helps your body's insulin and any diabetes medications do their job. If you are inactive or immobilized, the help your muscles can provide is reduced and your diabetes can worsen.

Certainly excess weight in younger age is a major player in the development of diabetes and if you are still in your 60s it's especially important to act now to reduce your chances of diabetes developing or worsening. Activity and exercise — particularly involving both aerobic and resistance strategies — will improve your diabetes control whether you lose weight in the process or not.

Diabetes is covered in greater detail in Chapter 6. Here it's sufficient to say that the same rule applies to people with or without diabetes, that is, do everything you can to boost your muscles and don't aim to lose weight by dieting alone.

WHAT ABOUT CALORIE RESTRICTION OR INTERMITTENT FASTING FOR A LONGER, HEALTHIER LIFE?

You may have read about or heard people speak of *calorie restriction*, and that *intermittent fasting* — not eating at all on one or more days a week, (included in the '5/2 plan' and similar diets) — can improve your health and also possibly extend your lifespan.

Calorie restriction bases its claims on scientific findings that if you under-feed experimental animals (i.e. feed fewer calories (kilojoules) than the animal would eat if food were available to them all day) for their entire adult lives, they live longer than those animals which are allowed to choose how much they eat.

Calorie restriction enthusiasts and some nutrition researchers believe the same applies to humans. There is research that shows that it may do so, and in a rural area in Japan where people eat according to the rule 'have only 80 percent of what you need to make you feel full', individuals commonly live healthy, active lives to well into their 100s. Researchers believe the strategy of restricting calories leads to this longevity. Of course those people also live relatively active, rural lives in smaller communities, which may play a part as well.

Whatever the reasons, it's a virtuous plan and maybe it *is* the answer to long life but one unavoidable fact remains: if you are already 65 or so IT IS TOO LATE TO START!

In order to be safe and effective, calorie restriction must be practised for as close to lifelong as possible (at least for most of an adult's life, i.e. 40 years or more). And during that time, food intake requires constant vigilance, a good under-standing of nutritional science and an active lifestyle in order to get full benefits.

For people already well into mature age — getting closer to 90 than 50 — who are not already avid calorie restriction adherents, this is definitely NOT the time to take it up. Unless you are also involved in a carefully designed exercise and nutrition program all that is likely to happen is that you will lose out on body muscle as well as nutrients.

Intermittent fasting has an increasing following and with good reason in younger people: it does seem that regularly challenging your body's physiology by having no food at all some days (or very limited amounts) can offer a number of health benefits into later life. Of course that is the way our forebears would have lived so maybe there is something in that. Whatever the reason, timing is everything. Cheating aging from now on relies on keeping up a good supply of protein, antioxidants and other nutrients and that's hard to do if you have to restrict what you eat some of the time.

For those of you who have very good nutritional knowledge and can plan a highly nutritious protein and nutrient-dense diet on your non-fasting days as well as keeping up a rigorous exercise schedule to avert muscle loss, then intermittent fasting may well be a good idea. But for most of you reading this, it's the same as calorie restriction: it's just too late to start.

Being 'a bit overweight' is better for your health than being very lean now

It's true. The science is quite clear: people beyond 65 or so, and who are a bit heavier, have fewer health problems and are likely to live longer than those who are thinner.

There are all sorts of guides for you to check where your weight, waist measurement and body fat fit so you can feel virtuous or devastated depending on the outcome. The BMI (Body Mass Index) is a common and easy one to use. But the 'healthy weight range' it identifies really applies when you are not yet in your seventies. This 'healthy weight' — whichever way you measure and compare it — is not about fashion, it's about the body weight that gives you the best chance of good health and longer life.

This is an area which has been under intense discussion worldwide among scientists and health authorities in the past few years and, while most now agree that the best BMI for older adults is better set at above 22, a new older age-specific guideline is yet to be published. This means that, what only a few years ago, may have labelled you as overweight (for example a BMI of 26), is now acceptable, while a BMI of 21, which would have been regarded as ideal for the younger you, now finds you too thin. The higher end of the ideal range is probably around 28.

If this seems strange to you, read on. It's partly about muscles, again, because muscle is heavier than body fat so if you lead an active life and are doing regular exercise you'll also have a higher BMI than someone less active. And because being more active is of course absolutely ideal for your health, so too is the higher BMI.

What's also possible is that heavier people are eating more food and thus getting more protein and anti-aging nutrients to help them out.

Whatever the reasons, the message remains: after 65 of age, it is no longer appropriate to consider dieting to lose weight and that being a bit cuddly is no longer a bad thing — in fact it's probably good for you.

SCIENCE SHOWS IT'S HEALTHIER TO CARRY A LITTLE EXTRA WEIGHT WHEN YOU ARE OLDER

Recent scientific studies of large numbers of older people found:

People already 70 to 75 years of age were 13 percent more likely to die in the following five years if they had a BMI in the 19 to 25 *range*, than if they had a BMI 25 to 30 (the former usually considered to be 'normal weight' for younger adults and the latter, 'overweight').[1]

Older women with a BMI *below* 22.5 and men below 23 (both classified in the mid range of 'normal' weight for younger adults) have more chance of experiencing ill health or dying compared to those with a BMI between 23 and 28.[2]

Nursing home residents, even those with a BMI that would put them in the obese range at a younger age (a BMI of more than 30), fared better health-wise than those who had a lower BMI.[3]

In a study of people aged 70 to 75 in Europe, the BMI at which people were least likely to die from any cause in the following 10 years was 27, a level considered overweight among younger adults.[4]

Irrespective of starting weight, in post-menopausal women an unintentional loss of as little as five percent of body weight in one year (that's only 3kg (7lb) if you weigh 60kg (132lb),, or 3.5kg if you are 70kg) is associated with increased risk of death in 5 to 10 years. It's likely to be similar for men.[5]

If elderly people are very lean they also suffer more complications in surgery than heavier people.[6]

1 Flicker, L et al. 2010 'Body Mass Index and Survival in Men and Women Aged 70 and 75', *Journal of the American Geriatric Association* vol. 58, no. 2, pp. 234-241.

2 Price, GM et al. 2006 'Weight, Shape and Mortality Risk in Older Persons: elevated waist-hip ratio, not high body mass index, is associated with a greater risk of death. *American Journal of Clinical Nutrition* vol. 84, pp 449-460.

3 Bahat, G et al. 2102 'Which Body Mass Index (BMI) is Better in the Elderly For Functional Status?' *Archives of Gerontology and Geriatrics* vol 54, no. 1, pp. 78-81.

4 DeHollander, EL et al 2012 'The Impact Of Body Mass Index in Old Age on Cause-Specific Mortality' *Journal of Nutrition, Health and Ageing* vol. 16, no.1, pp.100-106.

5 Diehr, P et al. 2008 'Weight, Mortality, years of Healthy Life and Active Life Expectancy in Older Adults' *Journals of the American Geriatrics Society* vol.56, pp76-83.

6 Miller SL & Wolfe, RR 2008 'The Danger of Weight Loss in the Elderly' *The Journal of Nutrition, Health and Aging* vol.12, no.7, pp. 487-491.

I am lean and active — surely that's the best isn't it?

Yes, it is best! The lifestyle choices you no doubt made many years ago that made you lean and active have prepared you for a long and productive life ahead. Keep your activities up and combine them with eating the right protein and nutrients to help your body and brain counter the effects of age, and you are set.

Constant vigilance is still essential: you must not lose weight. Your health can rapidly be impacted no matter how fit and well you are now. Even though you have a better muscle reserve than most, unintentional weight loss from now on will still include muscle and will quickly see you at below your ideal weight.

I have always been lean but don't need to exercise to stay that way — what about me?

If you are a lean person but are *not* very active and don't regularly do muscle-strengthening exercise then it might come as a surprise to learn that you are at *greater* risk from even a slight weight loss.

You may not have the risks to health that obesity imposes, and your lower weight has probably been a bonus in so many ways — including being the envy of most of your friends for years. But your muscle reserves will be less than those of a more active lean person, and may be even less than those of a heavier person so it won't take much to deplete your reserves if you should fall ill.

As well, if you have not had to exercise much to stay lean then you're probably only a small eater, which is not always a good thing from now on. If you have even a short time being off your food or if you cut down the amount you eat any more from now on, it's going to be much harder to get what you need to support your muscles.

It's just as well then that it's never too late to start doing the exercise your body needs.

And if you do find yourself struggling to eat well at any time, be sure to act quickly to boost the nutrition in every mouthful. The tips and ideas in Chapter 8 will help.

I'm not overweight but not under either — am I safe?

You are safe as long as you stay active and don't allow your weight to fall from now on.

If you lose any weight, you must consciously eat and work physically to rebuild as much muscle as you can, as soon as you can. It's too easy to accept becoming less and less active with age. You have earned a rest it's true but,

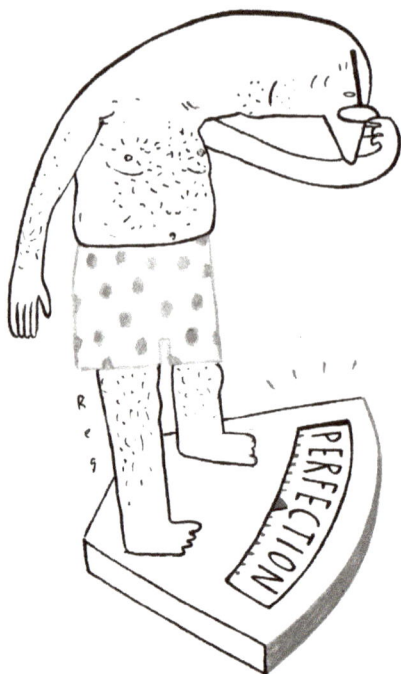

at 70 and with at least a decade ahead, eating and staying active will help those years contain the life you want them to.

But I feel like I'm getting fatter — there seems to be a belly I'm sure wasn't there before

It's sad but true that things *are* sliding southwards, some more than others. And one reason is that the bit of fat padding, which kindly fills out the wrinkles and keeps you rounded, gradually dwindles or might even change location. You can see it go most from your face and neck, your arms and legs, and all those disappearing bottoms are also evidence of the great southern journey. But annoyingly, it tends to hang on around your middle and some of the muscle you lose naturally with age does get replaced by fat, no matter what you do.

It's just not possible to do much about it diet-wise. You can keep muscle strong, and body fat at a healthy level but many healthy older people will still eventually adopt a more rounded body look with 'skinny' legs and arms. It doesn't necessarily mean you are piling on excessive fat kilos.

Even the most active among you may well have a bit of a belly. Your abdominal muscles are not as strong as they were, so even with not much extra body fat you are probably going to see that belly develop. If you prided yourself when younger on being lean you might struggle more than others to accept such changes. But it's vital that you do because dieting to lose your belly might put you at risk.

Even if you are carrying *a lot* of excess weight around your abdomen, which is widely thought not to be good for your health no matter what your age, the same applies: dieting to get rid of that now is counterproductive. Exercise of course is the key. Strengthening abdominal muscles and staying active to boost all your body muscle, while it may not completely get rid of that belly, is the only answer.

I have lost weight I didn't intend to lose — what should I do now?

It might not be possible now to regain all the weight or the muscle you've lost, but your independence depends on you giving it your very best try. And it's important to act before the situation gets worse.

That means eating enough to be able to rebuild muscle as well as putting anything you can back into storage. The rebuilding of course also needs you to do whatever activity you can and it's likely both the eating and the activity will be challenging.

To regain weight, particularly muscle, you need to eat more kilojoules (calories) and more protein. That doesn't mean you have to eat huge amounts of food but you do need to make even the smallest mouthful worth the effort. This is not 'normal healthy eating', it's a unique situation where most of the healthy eating advice you know gets turned on its head.

Sure, being active and getting all the exercise you need is ideal, but if you have lost weight through illness or an accident, then exercise might be a bit beyond your capabilities for a while. Make a start by eating properly first and add activity as soon as you can.

To regain weight what is needed now is more of a short term 'emergency' nutrition plan than anything resembling the advice elsewhere in this book. You need *extra* cheese sprinkled on pasta, extra butter melted over your vegetables, extra cream on your dessert, extra chips with your meal, extra milk powder added to your drinks. You need to choose the deep fried fish, not the grilled and to enjoy that tail on the lamb chop, not cut it off. Say 'yes' to the cake, the ice cream, the milkshake, the party pie and the crispy skin on the BBQ chicken. All these foods have plenty of kilojoules and many are also good suppliers of protein. And if you can't handle all that, try some of the high protein–high energy drinks and eating suggestions in Chapter 8 to help you.

If you need to boost your appetite you might need to apply a dual offensive, that is, tricks (covered in Chapter 3) along with strategies to make the most of what you can manage to eat (Eating Plan No. 3 in Chapter 8 will give you ideas).

Gerald's story

Gerald had been fairly active for most of his life and watched his weight but had gained about 10 or so kilos (22pounds) in his 60s. Then, after seeing a TV commercial for some diet shakes when he was 75, he decided to give them a go to lose those extra kilos.

He was very committed to the diet shakes and on some days even chose to have fewer than suggested. He lost 10 (22lb) kilos in only a month but even though he was now close to the weight he had been years before, just didn't feel as well as he had hoped.

His appetite was way down and while he thought this useful to stop him putting the weight back on, he was finding he had very little interest in food at all and could only eat very small meals. He continued to lose weight even though he no longer wanted to.

When his weight was down by 12 kilos (26lb), Gerald found that he wasn't able to do the things he wanted to. He had to bow out of a couple of bushwalks he was planning with friends because he just felt so tired and weak and was afraid he would fall or pass out on the walk. He began to find even getting out of bed in the mornings had become a challenge. Then he suffered a bladder infection and was very unwell, followed by a fall at home. He didn't break any bones fortunately but was stuck in an awkward position and couldn't get himself up until a neighbour happened to come by. He had a large cut on his leg and had to have community nurses come to dress that for many weeks while it very slowly healed.

Gerald found that his weight loss hadn't been good for him after all, and had hampered his independence.

What happened here?

Gerald was wrong to think that weight loss was a good idea at his age, especially such dramatic loss. It resulted in his appetite falling, in his rapid move into frailty and reduced his ability to heal and fight infection. Even though the diet shakes were probably high in protein, they were no doubt extremely low in calories. Not only that but, without carefully planned exercise to accompany his diet, Gerald would have lost a considerable amount of muscle and that quickly affected his health, his mobility and his independence.

Nothing stays the same: keep rethinking and updating

Everything you have read already in this book and will continue to do until the last page, needs to be considered in the context of the spring you have left in your step and how you are travelling.

You might find all this advice very interesting but know that it just doesn't apply to you if you are someone who wolfs down every morsel with relish and are too busy to *ever* sit still. But then again, if something unexpected thwarts your plans for a while you may suddenly find that 70 feels more like 90 than 50. Whatever's going on, it's essential that you continually rethink where you are in this book and adjust what you are eating accordingly.

The chances are that you are more likely to be one of the many for whom this might just be the time to relax a bit about what you think you should eat. The advice you took on in your 50s, or before — to avoid fat, cholesterol and sugar, to eat less meat, to drink only low fat dairy foods and never eat fried foods — was great for all sorts of reasons, not the least being to help you avoid piling on the kilos unnecessarily. But it needs a rethink as you move towards your 80s. Of course your choices now depend on everything we covered above, but low fat diets typically restrict some foods which supply vital nutrients in tasty packages. Cheese, for example, is a fabulous and delicious source of calcium and protein. Red meat is an excellent source of iron, zinc and selenium as well as protein. These are just two examples but there are plenty more covered in other chapters.

Live it up. Thin is no longer the pinnacle!

SUMMARY OF RISKS VS BENEFITS OF WEIGHT LOSS AT LATER AGE:

(particularly if more than five percent of original body weight is lost)

Risks from weight loss:

- You will lose strength
- A damaging fall is more likely
- You have a far higher chance of illness or infection
- Any illness or infection you do encounter will be harder to fight
- You will likely take longer to recover from any surgery
- You are likely to die sooner than someone who hasn't recently lost weight
- You are at higher risk of dementia (see Chapter 2)
- Without good exercise, your diabetes control may worsen

Benefits from weight loss

- Reduced strain on joints and organs
- Questionable (from current medical research) benefits to heart health or diabetes once you are in later age (unless weight loss is due to a combined exercise and food plan).

Chapter 6

DIABETES WHEN YOU ARE OLDER

If you have diabetes you'll be well aware that one size does not fit all. But as you move towards your later years one thing does apply to everyone: your diabetes management must also take account of the march of time. Whether you have had type 1 diabetes most of your life, developed type 2 many years ago or last month, whether you are very well rounded or *uber* lean and fit, it is pivotal in helping to make the most of the years ahead that you tailor your diabetes management to take into account the challenges your body faces in its later years.

Some of the cornerstones of your diabetes management up until now can actually cause harm in your later years, so need rethinking. When it comes to aging and independence, you are no different to every other older person: what you eat and do from now on — diabetes or not — can help you cheat aging, stay independent and let you live the life you had planned.

This chapter doesn't offer a complete guide to diabetes management; rather it gives an insight into ways you might need to adjust. Take the suggestions here and discuss them with your doctor and diabetes team so that, together, you can decide what suits your individual needs.

How to balance on a tightrope and juggle at the same time

Cheating aging vs what you need to manage your diabetes

Unfortunately, as you age, cheating aging *and* managing your diabetes don't line up as well as they did when you were younger.

A lot of diabetes management — especially when you are in your 40s, 50s and younger — is about reducing the chances you'll develop so called 'diabetes complications' over the years. And of course this is important, but some of the strategies can also be counterproductive when it comes to healthy aging in the years ahead: tight glucose control in particular might put you at higher health risk as you reach your later years.

Many people with type 2 diabetes also struggle to keep their weight down. There is no doubt that exercise and weight loss help avoid and treat this type of diabetes in younger people and exercise continues to be important no matter how old you are. But even with diabetes, weight loss at later age will do more harm than good unless it's carefully planned in conjunction with an appropriate exercise program.

Being overweight doesn't help diabetes, but any weight loss by dieting will mean muscle gets lost too. That worsens diabetes control and carries all the associated health negatives you've read about in previous chapters.

The big question: 'tight control' or not?

Tight control in diabetes means keeping the levels of glucose (blood sugar) in the blood close to the level of a person who doesn't have diabetes. Australian recommendations are under review but currently suggest blood glucose levels should be between 6 and 8 mmol/l (108-144mg/dl) before meals and 6 to 10 mmol/l (108 – 180mg/dl) two hours after starting a meal. (In New Zealand, USA and many other countries, the lower target is 4 or 5 (72 or 90) instead of 6, and Australia is likely to set similar levels in the review). That equates to an HbA1c (a test result familiar to most with diabetes and more commonly used in international circles to assess diabetes control) of below 7. These targets are necessary in young people because years of higher blood glucose levels can cause damage to the nerves and small blood vessels in the heart, kidneys, eyes and the limbs, especially the feet (producing diabetes complications) as well as affecting other body systems, including the brain.

To reduce your chances of these complications, tight control is the undisputed cornerstone of diabetes treatment when you are younger. But tight control *always* carries a risk that your blood glucose levels will fall below this target range now and then — into what is called hypoglycemia, or a 'hypo' (see the box here). For a younger person, the experience of a hypo is distressing but not usually dangerous. For a person in their later years, a hypo can be very dangerous.

A hypo hampers your brain's ability to coordinate body functions and makes you likely to fall — something which is well recognized as a potential disaster to your health and independence at later age. Suffering hypos regularly when you are older may also contribute to cognitive problems and will certainly reduce your confidence and ability to enjoy life.

Your chances of having a hypo in later age increase for three main reasons:

- Your ability to realize that your blood glucose levels are falling can fade as you become less able to recognize the signs and to act quickly enough to take evasive action.

- If you've had diabetes for some years a hypo can happen at a higher blood glucose level than it once did. So while 4 mmol/l (72 mg/dl) might have been your red light zone before, it could be 5 (90) or even higher for you now.

- And then there's what you eat. Reduced appetite and eating less than you need can have bigger consequences in diabetes. If you don't eat enough food — especially carbohydrates to keep blood glucose supplies up — then a hypo is on the cards.

Not everyone with diabetes is at risk of a hypo. People with type 2 diabetes controlled by diet alone or taking other types of oral medications are not at risk of a hypo. You are at risk if you have type 1 diabetes or if you have type 2 and are either injecting insulin or taking certain oral medications which 'push' your body to make extra insulin or assist insulin in other ways (see the list of medications here). If you are not sure, ask your doctor.

But even without a hypo risk, sometimes maintaining tight control means you limit the food you eat, whether you notice you are doing it or not. That makes it difficult to get the protein and other nutrients you need to face the challenges of age. A few years of not getting quite enough protein and other nutrients can affect your muscles, bones and brain surprisingly quickly.

Deciding if and when you need to relax diabetes control

Whether you need to relax your diabetes control is a very individual decision, and you must keep revisiting your requirements every year or so, and more often if you are unwell, or past 80. Relaxing control means allowing blood glucose levels to be a bit higher than previously, which means you avoid the chance of them falling low enough to cause a hypo, but as a consequence they will also rise higher than those you (and your doctor) may have been comfortable with in the past.

If you aim to always avoid blood glucose levels below 6 then they are also going to hit 15 or 16 (270-288 in mg/dl) at times and occasionally go higher.

Those upper levels would have been enough to elicit an audible gasp from your diabetes team in the past, but from now on may be essential for many of you.

Relaxed control has big advantages for some. It allows greater flexibility in what you eat, helps keep your appetite up if it's failing, lets you eat as well as you need to help your body confront the challenges of age and, most importantly, greatly reduces your chances of a hypo. And in later old age, if you are frail, a hypo can lead to stroke or a heart attack.

But relaxing control is not for everyone. If you are still in your 60s or 70s and quite well, then you have decades ahead and the benefits of tight control easily outweigh the risks of a hypo. As long as you eat according to the advice elsewhere in this book, you'll enjoy those years. You'll just need to regularly reassess how you are doing as you move into your 80s and beyond and possibly rethink employing tight control as time goes on.

The importance of exercise and how to plan for it with diabetes

Exercise is an extremely important part of diabetes management at any age, but can also trigger hypos in some people if your exercise is not adequately planned. That's because if you are on insulin or taking one of the medications listed below, adding exercise can bring your blood glucose levels down low enough to cause a hypo. But that's no reason at all to avoid exercise, all you need to do is add extra carbohydrate-containing snacks and drinks and, in some cases, adjust your insulin or other medication dose when you exercise. You need to discuss this with your diabetes team to develop a plan that's best for you. It's absolutely clear that whether you have type 1 or type 2 diabetes, if you are lean or overweight, exercise will improve your diabetes control, help you avoid complications and continue living the life you had hoped for.

Of course you must **always** check with your doctor before you start any strenuous exercise plan but don't allow yourself to become complacent, you might be able to achieve more than you thought you could and all of it will help you cheat aging.

SOME ORAL DIABETES MEDICATIONS THAT CAN CAUSE HYPOGLYCEMIA

Brand names are shown in italics and may vary depending on the country of purchase

Diamicron™, Glyade™, Diamicron MR™, Nidem ™

Daonil™, Semi Daonil™, Glimel ™

Glucovance™

Melizide™, Minidiab™

Amaryl™, Di mirel™

Novonorm™

Diabetes and your brain

Diabetes, it seems, may contribute to the development of dementia in some people. There is lots of research going on to check this out and to try to find exactly why this might be. There are no clear answers yet; it may come down to how well you have managed your diabetes over the years, it may be related to repeated hypos, it could be the way insulin affects brain cells themselves and it could even be the combined effect of a number of other players. Whatever it is, it's important to remember that it's not as black and white as may have been made out in the past: having diabetes is *not* a guarantee you will also get dementia, but it does seem glucose has effects in the brain that we haven't been completely aware of until quite recently.

From recent research, it seems high levels of blood glucose (even at the high end of the normal range) may also affect the brains of people without diabetes. That's a worry because you are not always going to know they are high until they rise enough to register as diabetes and by then they might already have had some ill effect.

But what is important to remember before you panic, is that everything already said about being active and eating to support your muscles and brain holds extra sway here. In fact, exercise is the ultimate weapon. Your muscles use up excess glucose as they work to keep blood levels in control so everything already said about activity — particularly resistance exercise — is key here too. Decreasing activity in daily life might even explain the presence of higher than ideal blood glucose levels.

Exercise might not be the complete answer but it's a big contributor at the very least, and it has so many spin-off benefits.

And don't forget — glucose is not a bad guy, your brain relies on it as its premium fuel source. But it needs just the right amount — not too little, not too much.

Food for thought

The pros and cons of 'tight control' in later age

It's not possible to give advice appropriate for each and every reader, but the following are suggestions applicable to many people living with diabetes. If you are not sure what's appropriate for you, discuss what you read here with your doctor or diabetes team.

If you are mostly well and have had diabetes since before your 60s

Whether you have type 1 or type 2 diabetes, it may be quite a while since you were diagnosed and, of course, you still have many years ahead. If you have developed complications they will affect your management but they shouldn't stop you remaining active and eating in the way you've read about in this book. To avoid any complications worsening and to reduce the chance of new problems cropping up, you should continue with the diabetes management strategies you already have in place but do review those strategies as you advance in age, or if you become unwell.

If you have had type 2 for many years, then you also need to consider the progress of your diabetes. Type 2 happens when your body can't produce all the insulin it needs to keep blood glucose at normal levels, but many people don't realize that it's usual for insulin production to continue to decline over the years. Even if your control has been excellent, your blood glucose levels will gradually rise, and require different management. Since diet has such an influence on those levels it's very common to assume that the gradual worsening of your blood sugar levels is because you have been eating badly. But it's not all about food, it's about the natural progression of type 2 diabetes and requires medical management. You may need to start medication if you haven't yet taken any, or to take extra medication, or to change to something different. If you just made changes to your diet to compensate, you are likely to eat less food and get less of the nutrients you need — something you just can't afford to do.

Exercise plays an important part too: being active and especially getting good resistance exercise slows this progression and assists in the management of your diabetes. The same exercises outlined in Chapter 2 are also great for diabetes as long as you discuss strategies for avoiding hypos with your diabetes team before you start anything new.

If diabetes has only been part of your picture since your early 60s and you are not yet in your 80s

If you are active and otherwise in good health the same applies for you as for someone diagnosed some years ago: tight control is important as long as you remain active, eat well and don't lose weight without appropriate exercise.

If you are not active and healthy, you may need a different focus. The ideal will be to do what you can to boost your activity levels and follow the eating advice elsewhere in this book. But if health issues limit your ability to do that, your diabetes may need to be treated as it would for someone considerably older because risks associated with suffering a hypo may just be too high.

If you have been diagnosed with type 2 diabetes only since your late 70s, 80s or even later

It's questionable whether the sort of diabetes which develops late in older age needs medical or dietary treatment at all. Diabetes at later age is a medical condition that is distinct from one diagnosed in younger people, but too often it's treated in the same way. The effects of the dwindling ability of your body to produce insulin combined with reduced body muscle mean that insulin production falls with age in *all* people so almost anyone who lives long enough can eventually develop blood glucose levels in the diabetes range. That doesn't mean they should always be treated with medication and it certainly doesn't mean it's time to cut down on the food you eat. Well meaning friends, family and even some health professionals might encourage you to reassess your diet but that needs to be done with great caution: any restriction on what you eat in later age, and its consequences in weight and muscle loss are just not worth the risks.

At later age, it's extremely important to discuss the risks with your doctor versus the benefits of medical treatment. Higher blood glucose levels can slow healing and have other effects, especially in blood circulation. That means glucose levels may need to be managed for some people, but for very many others they are not significant enough to require medical treatment. It's essential that you don't start limiting the food you eat because let's face it, although tight control prevents complications, they probably won't have time to develop significantly in the limited number of years ahead, so the benefit is debatable.

Again, the main thing worth considering is exercise: even if you are already at an advanced age, or are quite frail, anything you can do will be of benefit as long as it is first cleared by your doctor.

If you have lost weight, and have any type of diabetes

If you have lost weight over the past few years then that's a problem in itself: you've already read how damaging it can be, and how it also affects your diabetes control.

It's also easy to develop a vicious circle of weight loss, which results in muscle loss, which contributes to rising blood glucose levels. If you then try to eat less to bring the levels down, the situation worsens — more weight goes, with it more muscle goes and the circle continues.

This is something commonly seen in hospital: a frail person with diabetes who has been trying to keep their blood glucose levels down by eating less and less eventually loses so much weight and becomes so unwell they land in hospital. There they are soon found to be malnourished and well-meaning dietitians supply nutritious foods and snacks. As a result the patient's blood glucose levels skyrocket and the patient and hospital staff react with alarm. But it's not the food at fault — food is the essential treatment for malnutrition. The patient's medication needs looking at and a whole new plan for diabetes control worked out.

Weight loss and pre-diabetes symptoms

Weight loss can also reveal diabetes or pre-diabetes symptoms (raised blood glucose levels) in later age even in those who haven't previously had diabetes because it involves loss of muscle and thus reduces your ability to use excess blood glucose.

What you really need to do if you have been losing weight and experiencing rising blood glucose levels is eat *more* and to exercise, if you can, to stop any further loss and make up for the weight and muscle that's been lost.

Special considerations for people with diabetes:

Dealing with chronic renal (kidney) failure

If your kidneys have been affected by diabetes and you have been diagnosed with Chronic Kidney Disease (abbreviated as CKD but also called Chronic Renal Disease or Chronic Renal Failure) then, at some stage, you may need to reconsider your intake of protein and some other nutrients (especially potassium, phosphorous and salt). Kidneys can usually process any amount of protein waste, but if they are damaged by diabetes sometimes you need to eat less protein to help them cope.

Restricting protein of course goes against a lot of what has been recommended elsewhere in this book for optimal health as you age, so if your kidney specialist has told you to restrict your protein intake, you will need the advice of a dietitian to help you plan an appropriate diet.

The best protein for someone with kidney disease is high quality protein that comes from animal foods: all meats, chicken and poultry, fish and seafood, eggs and dairy foods.

You may also need extra kilojoules to avoid losing weight if your protein is just used up as fuel — that means adding extra cream, butter or oil, having fried foods and pastries and often having special supplement drinks formulated especially for those with kidney disease. This sort of individual advice needs to come from your dietitian otherwise it will be risky to know if you are eating what's best for you.

Frustratingly, one of the biggest problems which people with CKD face is muscle wasting. It happens as a consequence of CKD and significantly cuts your chances of living independently. That means you need to exercise at the same time as eating enough protein to maintain and boost your muscles without stressing your kidneys further.

WHAT IS HYPOGLYCEMIA?

Hypoglycaemia means low blood glucose, but it refers to blood glucose levels below what would normally occur in someone without diabetes. When your blood glucose falls low enough (usually below 4 mmol/l or 72mg/dl in most people) your brain function is affected and you have what's commonly called a hypo. As these levels fall you usually get a number of warnings that something is amiss — such as tingling in your face or arms and legs, vision changes, confusion, reduced coordination and a cold sweat. These warnings act as an alert and, as long as glucose is quickly supplied, levels rise out of this zone and you return to normal.

But if you are unaware they are falling (which can happen in some people and especially when you have had diabetes for many years) and glucose isn't supplied, then your brain becomes unable to keep you functioning and you suffer worsening of these symptoms and a loss of consciousness.

Chapter 7

YOUR DIET AND SURGICAL CUTS, CANCER AND CONSTIPATION

— special considerations for surgery —

Preparing for surgery

I am constantly amazed by the lack of discussion and awareness about the extra nutrition you need *before* and *after* any surgical procedure. Nutrition is so important at that time; your needs can be immense and yet are often completely overlooked.

If you are planning surgery of any kind, eating appropriately in the lead up as well as afterwards will help you come out of it the best you can. As with so many other things, this becomes more and more important as you get older.

It makes sense when you think about it, especially what you eat in the week or so before the operation. There is plenty of research evidence that shows boosting nutrition can minimize infection, increase the body's rate of repair and reduce the amount of time people have to spend in hospital. And you know what that means: you'll be back on your feet faster.

Boosting your nutrition is even more important if you end up with surgery as a result of an accident or sudden illness. That's because your body may also have extra demands placed on it by the widespread trauma from injury, inflammation or infection. Even more importantly, you will have had no opportunity to boost your nutrition beforehand. Eating well at such times can be the last thing you or even the medical staff might be considering, but it is absolutely essential if you plan to slot back into life where you left it.

Your body reacts to the assault of surgery by producing 'stress' hormones. These are important in helping your body cope but unfortunately cause additional muscle breakdown (and, remember, that's where your reserves of protein are stored). After any type of surgery you'll need many nutrients but protein is by far the most important because you'll be using huge amounts to repair and rebuild damaged tissue, fight infection and replenish lost blood. The bigger the surgery, the greater the needs, and if you do also suffer infection those needs skyrocket further.

Instead of being able to eat well at a time like this, you usually have to fast before the procedure then deal with a reduced appetite and limited intake afterwards. Without the protein from food, your muscle reserves have to supply what's needed and you may need three or four times the amount you would usually require, so that's an enormous drain on your muscles.

The older you are, it's little wonder you can struggle to recover from surgery, but if you consciously work at eating well and doing activities beforehand to boost your muscle reserves, your recovery will be quicker and the road to your ongoing independence will be much smoother.

So what do you need to do?

First and foremost, boost the amount of protein you eat in the lead up to your surgery and keep up whatever activity you can to support your muscles. Use the strategies for recovery from illness given in Chapter 1 and, foodwise, that means a protein food as the basis of three meals a day, plus an extra serve between meals.

For many people the best option is to add high protein drinks between or with meals. You can make them at home according to the recipes in Chapter 8, or buy any of the commercial supplements listed. Among them are some especially formulated for surgery patients. They contain particular amino acids (the building blocks of proteins) including glutamine and arginine and other nutrients considered to be especially useful.

You need to get something that suits you as well as your budget. Some supplements are quite costly but the less expensive, more widely available

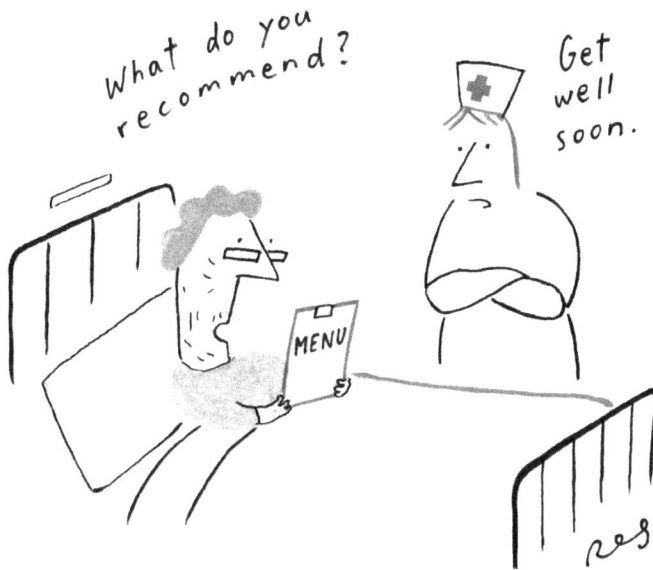

choices — or those made at home — are often just as effective. The worst option is if you do nothing.

This is not a time to be concerned about the possibility of gaining weight. This higher protein diet is a short-term prevention and recovery strategy. One week of higher protein intake before your hospitalisation may be enough for minor surgery; two weeks at least would be advisable for a major operation, especially if you aren't likely to return to normal eating directly after the procedure.

If you have lost weight in the lead up to your surgery then you may need more than that to make up for what's been lost as well as prepare you for what's ahead. In fact, if you have lost weight before planned surgery you should seriously consider whether you need to commit extra time rebuilding your muscle before you go ahead. Of course you can't put off life-saving surgery but heading into an elective operation with already depleted reserves is asking for trouble and may very likely hamper your recovery.

The nutrients you need to pay particular attention to apart from protein include:

zinc (wound repair)

iron (blood loss)

vitamin C (repair of damaged tissue)

as well as the antioxidants.

Commercial supplements contain a range of nutrients along with protein, so if you are using home made protein drinks you could add a general purpose multivitamin but, as always, check with your usual doctor that these are appropriate for you. If you are eating well, the additional vitamins and minerals probably won't be needed. It's protein that is critical at such times.

What about emergency surgery?

In all the flurry of medical activity, what you eat is too often forgotten but exactly the same applies as if your surgery is planned. You potentially face huge losses of protein from your muscles, and if you don't eat well that will escalate.

You can feel helpless as your medical and nursing team swing into action, but eating to aid your recovery is one thing you can take control of and do for yourself. Eat and eat well if that's possible — especially protein foods and as many colours as you can, or get supplements to boost your intake. You won't be able to stop some muscle loss, but you will be able to do a lot to slow that loss down and set yourself up for a faster recovery.

Unfortunately there isn't nearly enough focus in most hospitals on nutrition. Dietitians work hard to elevate its importance but budget constraints and lack of awareness of the issue too often don't allow the proactive menu planning which would help your recovery. That's a pity because, quite apart from the benefit to you in recovering faster, all sorts of costs to the health system can be cut if patients eat with recuperation in mind. If you heal more quickly, savings are made in wound care, in medications and in the length of time you need to remain in hospital.

But you can help yourself no matter what food is available by making sure you eat and if you can't face solid meals then there are often high protein supplements available as alternatives — ask the food service team or the dietitian. You can also have your own supply of supplement drinks and snacks brought in by friends or family if that's acceptable to the hospital

— just check with your doctor or the dietitian to be sure that what you are having is right for you.

I can't stress enough how important this is and you might have to take the initiative yourself if it's not suggested to you.

Diet and dealing with a cancer diagnosis

The information here is not about cancer prevention, there are many, many books on that. In part, it's about eating during cancer therapy, but more importantly, it's about how you can give your body the resources it needs in that confronting time of limbo which sits between your diagnosis or as tests are completed, and the time when your treatment starts.

You have to give your body all the resources it needs to support the cancer therapies ahead and at the same time ensure your chances of continued independence afterwards. To do that, you need to eat foods to help your body fight the cancer itself and minimize weight (especially muscle) loss so that doesn't eventually cause you further damage.

You will recall that a loss of enough body muscle is fatal in itself but you can do a lot to head this off before you start any treatment, as well as during the treatment phase.

And there is also no doubt that a 'never give up' positive attitude is crucial in the fight and this is certainly part of that strategy.

What to do right away

You can start right away to prepare for the assault of surgery, radiotherapy, chemotherapy or a combination of these. The same strategies which prepare you for elective surgery will work here but because you can't be sure exactly what's ahead it's worth adding a bit extra nutritional input. You need high protein, high kilojoule foods, supplements and meals and you should keep up whatever activity you can to help boost your muscles.

It's especially important to keep the variety of foods up — particularly boosting those multi-coloured vegetables, fruits and other foods that supply antioxidants. Don't forget, nutritionists believe it may be a combination of the antioxidants themselves with other components in these *complete* foods that provide the benefit, not tablets alone. (To refresh your memory, have a look at the more complete list of antioxidants in Chapter 4.)

You're going to get all sorts of advice on diets and supplements and it's common to be tempted by 'cleansing' diets or to cut out meat, dairy and other animal foods. To give your body the best chance to face what may be ahead this is not the time to start cutting these out. If you feel that diet changes will help you, then consider this only when your treatment is complete. Right now, you need those protein foods and the readily available nutrients like iron, zinc and vitamin B12. Focus on keeping your protein and energy up and add the colored foods for protection.

If you are already vegetarian or vegan that's different, you *should* already be getting the variety of colors but you must work to get the extra protein you need from nuts, seeds, soy foods, meat alternatives and pulses. That will mean larger amounts of plant protein foods and the addition of soy or other plant based liquid supplements if necessary.

And never forget that boosting your muscles and fully utilizing your protein intake, relies on your continuing to be as active as you possibly can. If you are already fit when you are diagnosed you probably have an advantage. Exercising or at least being active is also another thing you can do to help you boost muscle as well as helping you to feel positive.

What to do while you are being treated for cancer

Nowadays, cancer itself is frequently confounded and sent into remission as a result of advanced medical therapy and maximising the nutritional value of your food intake. But there is really no medical therapy that can stop the muscle loss that comes with cancer and is accelerated by any reduction in activity and eating.

Some cancer treatments are going to have you struggling to do even light exercise or eat anything at all. You'll also need a lot of rest to help you recover but take every opportunity to do whatever activity you can between rest periods and eat good high protein foods, even if it's only a few mouthfuls at a time. As soon as you feel better you can increase both.

If you can't cope with solid meals, then having a variety of high protein supplements and consuming as much as possible is a great idea. Use the suggestions in eating Plan 3 in Chapter 8. Juices can be a fantastic way to get in lots of antioxidants, cancer protective substances and vitamins, but they are low in protein. Adding a neutral flavor supplement or blending in nuts or seeds will supply protein and make a drink more like a smoothie.

The suggestions in Chapter 1 for recovery from illness also apply here.

It's undeniable that eating or undertaking activity when you are nauseous, when food often just doesn't stay down and when you feel sapped of energy is a huge challenge. But no matter what your treatment includes (surgery alone, or with radio or chemotherapy) anything you can do to hold onto and boost your muscle reserves will help you.

Beware of big claims

Beware of tablets or supplements with only one or two ingredients, no matter how good they sound. All the evidence suggests that different food components and nutrients work together better than they do individually. In large dosages, many food components, herbal preparations and even otherwise harmless substances can act completely differently to how they would if you got them from your food, and can even upset the actions of your cancer medications.

You *must* check everything you plan to take with your doctor or cancer team to be sure you won't cause yourself more harm than good.

Constipation

Again, this is a topic for a whole book in itself but it's such a big issue in older age it needs addressing here. It's an everyday problem for many people and is too often overlooked or given inadequate attention among the many different medical problems you may face.

Dealing with constipation is really important because not only does it make you feel miserable, it also reduces your appetite, often makes you feel nauseous, causes urinary incontinence and contributes to urinary tract infections.

Understanding how your digestion system works can help determine strategies to deal most effectively with constipation.

Your bowel is a long tube, narrow in the small intestine and wider in the large intestine. Food passes along the upper part in liquid form and water is gradually absorbed as the contents move along to produce a solid stool by the end. If food passes through the system too fast it will come out quite liquid (diarrhea) but if it moves too slowly it becomes dry and hard and thus difficult to move out. There are bands of muscle surrounding the bowel that contract rhythmically to push the contents along and those muscles work best when there is enough bulk for them to act on. The bulk comes from you eating plenty of food and from the contents being not too soft and not too hard. It's a bit like squeezing a toothpaste tube: when it's full it's easy to squeeze the toothpaste out, when empty it's much harder. If your intestine is mostly quite empty, with only occasional hard lumps, then those lumps can be more challenging for your muscles to push along, resulting in a slowing down and under-active system.

As you get older, your muscles can become less efficient and sometimes the nerves that coordinate their activity don't work as well so you don't perform as well in the bowel department as you once did.

It may be news to you, but your gut is a highly 'emotional' organ. Stress, grief, depression and many other emotional situations affect not just your mood but the functioning of other parts of your body too. Emotions can cause your bowels to speed up or slow down and the latter can contribute to constipation. It's possible that for some people with IBS (irritable bowel syndrome) this is part of the problem. (There are many great books available on IBS in bookshops to help you.)

For people who tend towards constipation from time to time, stress and worry can certainly make it worse.

In your abdomen, your large bowel (also called the colon) runs from your lower right side near your pelvis, up to just below your ribs, across to your left side then down to where it finally becomes the rectum where its contents are passed out. One common result of your bowels working too slowly or inefficiently is that gases, which are normally produced during food breakdown, accumulate instead of being moved along, causing not only flatulence but also gas build up higher in your bowel. Gas can get trapped anywhere along the colon causing bloating and a tight, swollen and often painful abdomen. In a chain reaction, when the gas builds up, the muscle bands can't work effectively and their rhythmic pulses are not able to push the gas or the solid contents along as well, worsening the problem. The longer the bowel contents stay inside you, the more gas gets produced, and the more water is removed from the stool, making it more difficult to pass through and causing extra discomfort.

One thing that can contribute to this is eating too little food. Your appetite is reduced when you are constipated but cutting down what you eat gives the intestinal muscles less bulk to help them do their work. Staying active and getting plenty of exercise will help move gas out, reduce the discomfort and help the contents move along as well.

'Overflow diarrhea'

One other thing that can happen in constipation is called 'overflow diarrhea'. That's when the bowel contents move so slowly that hard and quite dry masses of feces build up and are unable to be pushed along. They effectively block the bowel enough so that fluid builds up behind the large mass (though not enough to cause a bowel obstruction which is a medical emergency). Eventually, all this fluid either seeps past and flows out or can gush out suddenly. You often don't get a warning, which can be extremely distressing and embarrassing. It's also confusing because it seems like you have diarrhoea but it's actually constipation. The way to avoid this is to keep the bowel contents moving along.

The effect of medications on constipation

The side effects of medication are often the cause of bowel issues in older age because many commonly used medications contribute to constipation. Check the list at the end of this chapter but discuss any problems you are having with your doctor.

Some medications affect the action of the bowel, others change the absorption of water from the stool. Antibiotics reduce the number of bowel bacteria and, since around a third of the content of the stool is normally bacteria, that reduces bulk and makes it more challenging to move contents along. If you have taken antibiotics, a course of probiotics when your antibiotics are finished (tablets, yoghurt or drinks containing live bacteria cultures) can rebalance essential gut bacteria and help reverse the problem.

There are of course many medications to treat constipation. They work in three main ways:

> by keeping liquid in the stool (stool softeners)
> by speeding up the rate that food passes thought the bowel (bowel stimulants)
> by increasing the bulk of the stool (bulking agents and fibre supplements)
> or by a combination of these.

You need to work with your doctor to get the dose right though as some medications to treat constipation can go too far and then cause diarrhoea.

Something else to be aware of, is that iron and calcium supplements can also contribute — not when these vital nutrients come from food (iron especially from meats and calcium from dairy foods) — but when they are taken as tablets.

The good and the bad of fibre

The most common nutritional strategy for constipation is that you get plenty of fibre. Fibre is a bulking agent and does two things: it absorbs water and holds it, adding bulk to the stool and keeping the bowel contents soft. Adding fibre means you also need extra liquids. Often people cut down on fluids to try to avoid having to pass urine as frequently but, if you don't get enough fluid, that makes constipation more likely.

Fibre also encourages the growth of the healthy bacteria in your bowel, which helps too.

There are two problems which can crop up with fibre in older age: one is that many foods containing fibre are bulky and tend to fill you up before you get a chance to eat all the protein and other nutrients you need. And, with the exception of pulses like lentils, soybeans and the like, they contain little or no protein themselves. As you've already read, protein and antioxidants need to be your main food focus. Luckily many antioxidant foods are also fibre foods — think pulses, wholemeal and wholegrain breads, cereals and grains, fruits (especially dried), vegetables and nuts.

If you can only eat small amounts, then getting enough bulky high fibre foods can be difficult and that's where fibre supplements can help. There are a number of options: bran, psyllium and similar products can be sprinkled over cereals and meals or mixed into a smoothie. Commercial fibre powders, including the brands *Benefibre* and *Metamucil*, come flavored or unflavored and are mixed with water or other liquids. The benefit of the unflavored varieties is that they can be mixed into high protein drinks, soups and juices. The very commonly prescribed *Movicol* is a mix of fibre with a bowel stimulant.

When you add extra fibre you need to give your system time to get used to the change or it may cause excess gas build-up and discomfort. Start with a small change and if you are using a fibre supplement start with as little as a teaspoon a day and build up according to your doctor's advice or the instruction on the container until it's working. And then you need to stick with it so the problem doesn't start up again.

Because fibre can reduce the absorption of some minerals, including calcium, iron and magnesium, you need to be sure to get plenty of these if you are taking fibre supplements over the long term.

The other issue for some people is that adding more high-fibre foods results in extra gas build-up causing pain and distress without the benefit of reducing constipation. If, every time you try to increase your fibre, you get extremely bloated and uncomfortable then there are two things you can do. Firstly, try increasing your fibre *very* gradually. It may be easier to do that using psyllium or a commercial fibre supplement because you can easily vary the amount you use, or add small amounts of high fibre foods at a time. And secondly, you can try adding some probiotics. Adding good bacteria can help your bowels cope with the fibre and boost the volume of your stool, but take it gradually. And don't forget to keep your liquids up.

If these issues affect you, consult a dietitian to help you plan a food intake.

If you experience gas and bloating you may need to adopt a strategy of avoiding very high fibre foods, such as those in the top of the list here or at least avoid having more than one high fibre food at a time. It's not usually a strategy that would apply if you were much younger but may be necessary to help you manage symptoms in older age.

HIGH FIBRE FOODS

Wheat bran

High fibre breakfast cereals (usually bran based)

Rice and oat bran

Dried figs and other dried fruits

Legumes/pulses (dried peas, beans, lentils etc.)

Nuts and seeds

Wholemeal/wholegrain foods and breads

Vegetables — especially kale, cabbage, root vegetables, peas, corn, broccoli

Constipation is such a complex condition it's very difficult to provide a complete range of solutions here, but the following strategies will help most of us keep our bowels moving:

- Stay active and get plenty exercise. This is absolutely essential as the muscles in your abdomen and around your pelvis work as you exercise and as you move around and help push the bowel contents along. In fact just taking up a good walking and activity program may be all you need to reverse worrying constipation. It's also the way to help move any accumulated gases along and out and, sure, farting may be a bit antisocial but if you don't get those gases out they will just cause pain and you don't need that. Just pick an appropriate moment, along the same idea that if a tree falls in the forest and no one hears it, did it really fall?

- Eat! Your bowels need volume.

- Add extra higher fibre foods or supplements if you need to.

- Avoid dehydration. If you don't drink enough fluid that will make the stool harder.

- Be aware of the effect of medications and check the list below. If you are prescribed an opioid for pain (codeine, morphine, pain patches such as *Norspan* and *Durogesic*) then you will usually need a laxative to balance its effect. Many over-the-counter medications, including most cold and flu medicines and many pain relievers, contain codeine (have a look at the list here). If you are prone to constipation try to avoid these pain relievers but if you do have to take them, be prepared for your bowels to take a few days to return to normal.

- Be aware of the effect of antibiotics. While they are great at killing off bacteria that cause disease, they also kill off the good bacteria in the gut that help you process foods and keep your bowel healthy. As a result antibiotics can cause diarrhea and it takes a while for your good bacteria to recolonize. Probiotic tablets, powders or yoghurts containing good gut bacteria can assist as soon as you are finished the antibiotics.

MEDICATIONS COMMONLY ASSOCIATED WITH CONSTIPATION

(brand names may vary depending on the country of purchase)

The opioids	codeine (marketed as *Codeine,* also *Aspalgin, Codis, Codral, Codalgin, Mersyndol,* in many cold and flu medications)
	morphine (*Anamorph, MS Contin, MS Mono, Kapanol*)
	oxycodone (*Endone, Oxynorm, Oxycontin*)
	tramadol (*Tramal*)
	pethidine (*Parnate, Nardil*)
Some antidepressants	the TCAs (including *Tryptanol, Allegron, Endep, Tolerade, Tofranil*)
Some cardiac/blood pressure medications	verapamil (including *Verecaps, Anpec, Isoptin, Cordilox*), diltiazem (*Cardizem*)
	nifedipine (*Adalat, Adapine, Nifecard, Adefin Procardia*)
Some anticonvulsants	phenytoin (*Dilantin*)
	carbamazapine (*Tegretol*)
Iron supplements	many varieties
The NSAIDs (non steroidal anti inflammatory)	including ibuprophen (*Nurofen*) see also the lists of NSAIDs in Chapter 2

Chapter 8

THREE EATING PLANS
Tailored to you age, health and lifestyle

The aim of the plans in this chapter is not to restrict foods but to suggest the best options for your health and life stage.

What is common to all is that the main aim is *not* losing weight.

In Plan 1 it's also important to avoid *gaining* weight, but it's not designed as a weight loss plan because, if you need to lose weight in older age, exercise must be an integral part of your plan. You need to seek individual professional advice from a dietitian as well as an exercise professional to avoid the potential health issues that come with weight loss in older age.

Choose the plan that suits your stage of life and always vary the foods you eat.

'Variety's the very spice of life, that gives it all its flavor.'
—*William Cowper*

Plan 1

For those who are mainly in good health and haven't *unintentionally* lost weight

This is a guide to the sorts of foods you should include at each meal to help your muscles and brain and *relies on you doing exercise*. If you are not active then you need to find ways to become so. You *must work* to build and maintain muscle at the same time as eating.

The list here has a selection of protein-containing and other foods from which you can choose your own meals. You need to balance activity with what you eat to avoid gaining weight, or get additional advice from a dietitian.

If you have low appetite days or are not feeling 100 percent you may need to eat according to Plan 2 or 3, at least for a while. At such times it's fine to have:

- high protein drinks instead of a meal

- or just to eat desserts as long as they are higher protein desserts

- or just soups provided they are higher protein soups

- or even tea and toast for a short while, but you must have cheese or peanut butter, an egg or another protein with the toast

FOOD SELECTIONS: Plan 1

Breakfast options

Essential protein part of the meal	Eggs cooked any way
	Lean bacon, ham, breakfast steak or sausage
	Cheese (on toast) — can be grilled, or spread thickly with soft cheese (ricotta or soft goats cheese)
	Baked beans (on toast)
	(Toast with) peanut or other nut butter
	Commercial breakfast cereal with high protein milk or with added nuts, LSA* mix added for protein
	Nuts of any variety.
	Tofu or other soy product or meat alternative
	(*LSA mix is a blend of linseeds, sunflower seeds and ground almonds. It's high in protein and good fats as well as fibre.)
Fuel and antioxidant options to accompany protein	Tomatoes, mushrooms, spinach, any vegetables
	Fruit or dried fruit.
	Add as many different types of fruit, vegetables and grain foods as you need.

Main meal options

The same foods are appropriate for either the midday or evening meal.

Protein	Meat, egg, cheese, fish, tofu, lentils or other pulses, nuts, rice (when combined with nuts), pulses or soy protein (such as tofu).
Additions	Vegetables, salad, or a selection of salad vegetables in a sandwich — use as many different ones as possible
	Bread, rice or pasta
	Fruit.

Snacks

Snacks are not essential in this plan but if you are active and not gaining or losing weight then include them if you wish. If you need to avoid gaining weight then don't include snacks.

Higher protein options	Yoghurt, custard or similar dairy snack
	Cheese and crackers
	Nuts (or nuts and dried fruit)
	Fruit with cheese
	Sliced meats.
Antioxidant options	Fruit or dried fruit, fruit juice or fruit and vegetable juice
	Biscuits, cakes, etc. that incorporate fruit or vegetables and wholegrains.
	Fruit toast.

Plan 2

For those who have recently and unintentionally lost weight but still have a good appetite

This plan is designed to give you extra kilojoules as well as the protein and other nutrients you need.

You no longer need to choose all low fat foods so buy full cream milk, yoghurt and dairy foods (it's only three to four percent fat anyway), trim your meat only of thick layers of fat, choose a quality margarine or butter. Keep milk powder or a high protein supplement in the pantry to make high protein milk, yoghurt and soups, etc.

You should either eat three good meals a day, or three smaller meals with snacks in between. You need to try to keep your weight stable and if you regain what you've lost that's a bonus. Weigh yourself only once a week, or once every four days at the most to see how you're going. If you continue to lose weight move onto Plan 3, at least for a while.

If you are feeling unwell or not up to eating full meals, or if you don't fancy standard meals, you can choose to eat desserts or have soups or smoothies instead *as long as they are high protein*. You can have six to eight good snacks a day instead of meals. It doesn't matter which choice you make as long as they give you what you need.

FOOD SELECTIONS: Plan 2

Breakfast

Cereal or porridge with high protein (full cream) milk

Eggs cooked any way you like them with toast and bacon or other accompaniment. Spread your toast thickly with butter or an alternative spread. If you scramble your eggs use the recipe for high energy scrambled eggs

Fruit smoothie or milkshake made from the high protein drinks (see recipe list)

Bacon, ham, other meat or vegetarian alternative with any accompaniment

Baked beans or similar on toast. Enjoy your butter spread thickly

Cheese on toast — use thick cheese slices on wholegrain or wholemeal bread, with tomato or other herbs or vegetables as desired or have ricotta or similar soft cheese

Fruit with high protein yoghurt (see recipe)

Rice or noodle dish with meat, cheese or nuts added

Main meals	Meat, fish, seafood, chicken, egg or other animal protein
	OR vegetarian protein food (pulses, soybeans or soy based product, nuts, seeds)
	WITH any vegetable, salad or fruit accompaniment and rice or grain food
	Pasta, rice or bread may be added to any choice
	If you are struggling to eat adequate meals, boost what's in the meals you can eat: sprinkle a little cheese or chopped ham slices over vegetables or add cheese or nuts to a salad, melt butter over hot vegetables, add cheese sauce to dishes, add high energy gravy to meats (see recipes).
	You can use high protein drinks either between meals or as alternatives to meals if you need to. Choose a commercial supplement or make one from the recipes at the end of this chapter.
Add a dessert	If you have had a good protein food in your main meal then dessert can be anything you fancy. But if you were not able to eat a good main meal then dessert needs to supply your protein. Choose a high protein dessert from the recipe section.
Snacks	Snacks are useful in this plan if you are not able to eat well at each meal and are especially important if you are still struggling to keep your weight up. Many of the suggestions in Plan 3 are useful if you have lost weight but are not essential if your weight has stabilized. Where possible use snacks to boost your antioxidant intake.

Plan 3

For those who have lost weight and are struggling with a reduced appetite

This plan is not 'normal eating', it's an emergency rehabilitation plan to avoid further weight loss and to halt your rapid loss of independence. If you have become frail and continue to struggle to eat it is perfectly suitable to eat this way for the rest of your life if necessary.

It doesn't matters if you don't eat regular meals any more, have desserts all day or even eat the same food every meal as long as it gives you the protein, kilojoules and other nutrients you need.

I haven't divided this list into meals because you can choose any food from the suggestions here. Start with six to eight small portions of any food here if you can manage it. Again, you need to weigh yourself about every four days, or once a week is ideal.

Try to eat about every two to three hours. Have small amounts at first, even a spoonful at a time until you can handle more.

The foods in Plan 3 are all high in kilojoules but you're not likely to gain enough weight for that to be a problem. When your weight stabilizes you can move onto Plan 2.

You will need to stock your pantry or fridge with items from the shopping list.

SHOPPING LIST: Plan 3

High protein supplement powders

There are many varieties on the market. Check with your pharmacist and pharmacy outlets. The supermarket brands generally don't contain the same range of nutrients. There are two Australian made products: *Enprocal* powder, a neutral flavor for sweet or savory foods; and *Proform*, available in neutral, vanilla and chocolate. *Sustagen (Nestle)* and *Ensure (Abbott)* are the most commonly known alternatives. *Sustagen* is now available unflavored as well as the better known vanilla and chocolate flavors. *Ensure* is vanilla flavored and is lactose free.

There are also a number of vegan and vegetarian powders available, mostly from health food stores, online or from pharmacies.

Whey based powders

Whey is a by-product of cheese production and has been shown to be especially good at improving muscle function in older people. Whey is quite costly, especially the whey protein isolate, which is the most concentrated, but has shown good results for some older people.

Soy protein isolate is a similar product suitable for vegans.

Body-building powders

These are usually similar to the powders above and are sold in gyms and healthfood stores but it's best to check with your doctor or dietitian first to be sure they are okay for you.

Milk powder or skim milk powder

These can be substituted for the protein powders (see above) as their protein content is similar. They cost less but don't contain the range of micronutrients that the more popular commercial supplements do. Full-cream milk powder is not as high in protein as skim milk powder but has extra calories and imparts a richer flavor. Either are suitable.

Cheese: cheddar or soft cheeses of any variety	Ready sliced, cubed or grated cheese, packaged wedges, small portions or cheese sticks (often used for kids' school lunches) are useful to have on hand.
Sliced meats or barbecued chicken	Store these in the fridge immediately and throw out any not used after 48 hours.
Ready-to-heat frozen snack foods	Suggestions include party pies, sausage rolls, samosas, chicken drumettes or nuggets, mini quiches, fish cocktails and fish pieces, fish-in-sauce.
Ready-made meals	Try to avoid low fat and 'diet' varieties (but, if you buy these, add grated cheese, cream, butter or high protein gravy during reheating to boost their kilojoules), pies and quiches.
Gravy powder or ready-made gravy and sauces	
Yoghurt	Preferably NOT low fat. You need to look for any that are made using full cream milk. Many of the gourmet yoghurts are not low fat, nor are most Greek-style yoghurts.
Other dairy desserts: custards, mousse, crème caramel	*Avoid* low fat if possible, but you can always add cream at home.
Cream	Fresh or buy UHT cream to store in the pantry.
Paté	Those made from chicken liver, meat or smoked fish.
Icecream tubs, mini icecreams	The best are gourmet icecreams that are usually higher in fat but any will do.
Canned or microwaveable dessert puddings	
Soups of any variety including cup-of-soups	Prepare with milk powder or neutral flavored high protein supplement powder to boost their nutrition.
Small cans of tuna, salmon or any sort of meat (chicken is now also widely available)	
Small cans of baked beans	Baked beans are higher in protein than canned spaghetti.

MEAL OR SNACK OPTIONS: Plan 3

Choose at least six to eight of these per day

Commercial supplement drink	made to directions
Milkshake or smoothie	from recipes
High protein fruit, vegetable juice or fruit and vegetable smoothie	from recipes
Iced coffee with or without sweetening	from recipes
High protein yoghurt	yoghurt or custard with a heaped dessertspoon of high protein supplement powder (neutral flavor or vanilla) or milk powder
Fruit with high protein yoghurt	
Cup-of-soups (or pre-made soup)	with one or two heaped dessertspoons of high protein supplement (neutral) or milk powder added
Any of your frozen snack foods	reheated
Scrambled egg or boiled egg	A hard boiled egg with mayonnaise is another good option
Egg, cheese or meat sandwich	with a salad preferably
Cheese with crackers or sticks of celery, carrot or apple	
Paté and crackers or toast	
Peanut butter on toast	
Cheese or baked beans on toast	
Icecream	with a heaped spoonful of a flavored high protein supplement powder (vanilla or chocolate) or sprinkled with chocolate drink powder (*Milo, Ovaltine, Akta-Vite,* etc.)

Handful of nuts or nuts and dried fruit	
A couple of slices of cold meat or a piece of cold barbecued chicken	
A big spoonful of peanut butter	right from the jar!
Commercial ready-made meal	and if they are diet or low fat meals, add cheese for extra protein and cream for calories
Breakfast cereal or porridge	sprinkled with a heaped spoonful of a vanilla or other flavored high protein supplement powder
Any vegetable or meat with cheese or mornay sauce	
A small can of tuna, salmon or chicken	
Commercial snack bars based on nuts or marketed as high protein	these are good emergency options but many are low fat and sugar free so they're not always ideal.

Sandwich tips

- There is *no* need to avoid butter or margarine. You may put a generous spread on your bread.

- In place of butter or margarine, or even in addition, use cream cheese or cheese spread to boost the protein content of your sandwich.

- If a whole sandwich is too much, just have one slice of bread but fill it well.

- If you are having cold meat, have at least two slices, not just one.

- Add sliced or grated cheese to as many sandwiches as you can. Salad or tomato is great but the cheese will add protein and calcium too.

- Peanut butter or other nut butters are great protein foods for sandwiches.

- If you want a sweet sandwich then have one — jam or honey is great — but spread the bread with cream cheese rather than butter to boost the protein and calcium content of your meal.

- As an indulgence, spread your bread with butter, then sprinkle a spoonful of Milo or similar powdered drink on your sandwich.

If you are having problems swallowing foods

Swallowing problems are common in elderly people and can, unfortunately, cause chest infections and further weight loss.

You need to speak with your doctor if you are having any problems swallowing your food or if you are coughing or have a raspy, gurgly chest (not gurgling in your stomach, but in your chest) after eating.

You may need the help of a speech pathologist; they deal with swallowing issues as well as speech.

Sometimes it can be as easy as just making sure the food you eat is not too dry by adding extra gravy or sauce to your meals, choosing casseroles or soups. You can also avoid dry meats, toast or foods like crisps that can easily get stuck if your swallowing is poor.

If you are struggling with nausea

Nausea can be caused by many things as you have read previously in Chapter 2, but not eating or drinking well is a big factor. It's difficult when you feel ill but try to have small amounts of food often — even a teaspoon at a time — till the nausea abates. Check the options suggested in the previous chapter.

If it doesn't stop, speak with your doctor for other options.

It *is* possible to turn weight loss around

You can avoid further decline, and also regain some of what has been lost.

It will take a concerted effort.

It will take you ignoring any mistaken appetite cues to achieve an appreciable return to health and continued independence.

It will take an exercise program that you can safely manage.

Exercise is essential to encourage any possible rebuilding of muscle. It really needs professional involvement, ideally a physiotherapist or an exercise physiologist, who will design a specific program for you to rebuild muscle and to avoid causing harm.

If that's too costly, look out for community run programs. There are a variety of excellent exercise programs available for older people. Tai chi and similar exercise is fabulous for balance and core strength. The exercises suggested in Chapter 1 are all great but, of course, any new exercise plan must be discussed with your doctor first.

RECIPE IDEAS

High protein cold drinks

High protein milk

- 1 litre (2 pints) full cream milk (just remove enough from a carton to add the powder
- 1 cup skim milk powder, full cream milk powder or unflavored protein supplement powder

Sprinkle powder over milk and mix. Store in the fridge as you would regular milk.

It's best to get a jug with a lid that will hold more than a litre then mix the high protein milk and keep in the fridge. Alternatively, mix the high protein milk and return to the carton. Use this for all drinks and recipes.

High protein milkshake

Makes 1 serve

- 200ml (7 oz) full cream milk
- 2 tablespoons high protein supplement powder
- Flavoring to taste

Blend and keep any leftover in the fridge for no more than 24 hours

High protein fruit smoothie

- 200ml (7 oz) full cream milk
- 2 tablespoons high protein supplement powder
- 1 piece of fruit or half a cup of berries (peeled or seeded as necessary)
- Sugar or honey to taste if required

Blend in a food processor till fruit is thoroughly combined. Store any leftover in the fridge for less than 24 hours.

High protein green boost drink

- 200ml (7 oz) juice or milk
- Handful of kale or similar leafy green vegetable
- Small handful of raw nuts such as almonds
- 1 tablespoon of unflavored high protein supplement powder
- Sugar or honey to taste

Blend in a food processor until thoroughly mixed. Store any leftover in the fridge for no more than 24 hours.

High protein hot drinks

Note that most high protein supplements will curdle if boiled or made with boiling water so always add powders *after* first heating other ingredients.

High protein coffee, tea or chai

Either use high protein milk in these or add 1 to 2 tablespoons of powdered supplement or milk powder to your drink.

Make coffee with high protein milk instead of water.

Milo, Horlicks, Ovaltine or similar

These powders are all good protein sources – make them with high protein or regular milk.

Cup of soup or home-made soup

Make according to your recipe or packet directions then cool slightly and add 2 tablespoons of skim milk powder or neutral flavor protein supplement per person after

Other high protein recipes

High protein breakfast options

Use high protein milk on your cereal or sprinkle vanilla flavored supplement powder on top of your cereal or porridge.

When making porridge, slightly cool the porridge then add 2 tablespoons of skim milk powder or unflavored protein supplement per person.

Add 1 tablespoon of skim milk powder to your mix for scrambled eggs before they are cooked, or melt cheese in after cooking the eggs.

High protein gravy

Make up gravy mix with hot or boiling water according to directions, cool slightly

Add 2 tablespoons of skim milk powder or neutral flavor protein supplement per person.

For use in a casserole, add 2 tablespoons of skim milk powder or neutral flavor protein supplement per person to warmed (but not boiling) liquid stock. Add this to a pre-cooked casserole just before serving.

High protein custard or dairy dessert

Make custard according to directions then remove from heat, cool a little and stir in 2 tablespoons of skim milk powder or unflavored protein supplement per person.

High protein jelly

This will make an opaque dessert, rather than clear jelly but the taste is similar and less milky than custard.

Make jelly according to directions then cool slightly and add 2 tablespoons of skim milk powder or neutral flavor protein supplement per person. Whisk until dissolved and allow to set as usual.

High protein biscuits, cake or pikelets

Make according to your usual recipe adding 2 tablespoons of skim milk powder or unflavored protein supplement per person to the flour before mixing it in. Cook as usual.

Additional recipe ideas

Any of the **(unflavored) supplement powders or milk powder** can be added to mashed potato: use 2 tablespoons per person as a guide.

Ground nuts or seeds (including LSA mix — a blend of linseed or flax seeds, sunflower seeds and almonds) make great high protein as well as high fibre additives into drinks and even baked goods and casseroles. Add about 1 to 2 tablespoons per person.

You can add fibre to casseroles and soups by adding 1 to 2 tablespoons (per person) of **lentils or beans** (lima, cannellini, kidney etc.) during cooking.

Similarly, add about 1 to 2 tablespoons of **wheat, oat or rice bran** to cakes and any baked goods to boost fibre. Cakes, slices and biscuits made using **dried fruits and nuts** also have extra fibre.

Appendix

MOVE IT, DON'T LOSE IT
Exercise and Activity Tips

All activity at later age should be discussed with your doctor and is best done with the assistance of a qualified exercise professional.

These additional guidelines are to give you an idea of what will be of most assistance in muscle maintenance and rebuilding strength after illness or time spent in bed.

First,

- always warm up and cool down for at least five minutes either side of exercise
- walk or do light movements of the muscle areas you are planning to work

and a few words of caution:

- don't exercise if you are ill. It's okay if you are recovering from an accident or surgery and are able to do some exercises, but not if you are actually suffering an illness
- build up all activity gradually
- you should expect to feel mild muscle soreness in the days after exercise but as you get used to each activity that will fade. Any severe pain means stopping that exercise and needs to be checked with your doctor, physiotherapist or professionally qualified exercise professional.

Next,

Plan your exercises!

To avoid overuse causing you excess pain use different muscle groups on different days. It's best to plan to use one or two major muscle groups each time you do strength exercises especially. Then after a couple of days, work a different group. Allow at least a few days between repeating an activity in the same muscle group.

Aerobic activities like walking, jogging, cycling, swimming and sport activities use a wide range of muscles and won't usually require these considerations, though you do have to work up the length of time you spend on each.

Resistance bands and weights

Resistance bands are flexible elasticized bands that are wrapped round your hands while you do activities to help you work against the resistance they present. Your exercise professional can instruct you how to use them.

You can purchase 500g or 1kg hand or ankle weights (or heavier) but you can also use everyday items such as cans of soup or even bags of shopping.

With both, its essential to start slowly at the lowest weight you need. For some people, that may be no weight at all at first, then working up to heavier weights as you progress.

To be assured you are gaining benefit, each activity should feel challenging and even a bit hard.

The weight is too heavy if you can't repeat the exercise eight times and you should then drop back in weight until your muscles have become accustomed to the lower weight first.

Aim to be able to repeat each exercise 10 to 15 times. When you can do those easily you can add more weight if you wish and are able.

Don't move too fast and don't quickly drop your weights. A rule of thumb is to count to three as you lift, push or pull; hold for one count then take two counts to return to rest.

Always breathe out as you lift, push or pull, and breathe in as you return to rest.

Resources to help your exercise plan

Exercise suggestions are available in many books and resources.

www.activeageingaustralia.com.au (telephone 08 8362 5599) produces a good home exercising book and DVD to give you additional guidance on exercises and intensities

www.healthinsite.gov.au/article/physical-activity-guidelines-older-adults has good information and suggestions on appropriate physical activities, although the nutrition guidelines on the same website need updating for older people — they don't yet align with the latest scientific thinking and the guidelines in this book.

COTA (Council on the Ageing) in your state may also have useful information on accessing programs and activities for strength and activity training. In South Australia the Strength for Life program is especially good and anyone can access resources from this program at **www.cotasa.org.au.**

Most health departments and many local councils also have resources you can access.

www.cdc.gov/physicalactivity/growingstronger is an American site (US Centre for Disease Control) that has excellent information.

Nutrition Supplements

It's always best to ask your dietitian about which nutritional supplements might be best for you.

Below is a list of companies that produce commercially available nutritional supplements you can purchase without the need for a prescription.

Many are available or can be ordered from your local pharmacy or, alternatively, can be purchased online, often at a lower cost. The Paraplegic and Quadriplegic Association of Australia runs an excellent online shop called BrightSky (**www.brightsky.com.au**) supplying a wide range of healthcare needs to practitioners and the public. Look on this website under nutritional support then oral supplements for products. You can order online or over the phone and they deliver to your home.

Compare prices as they can vary a lot.

Always remember that if you need a nutritional supplement, it can provide excellent nutrition in place of meals and although many supplements may seem costly if compared to a soft drink or a flavored milk, when you think of them of as replacing a complete meal they are very cost effective.

AUSTRALIAN SUPPLEMENT PRODUCERS

www.proformonline.com.au or 1300 362 774 (aust)	*Proform* powder (unflavored, vanilla or white chocolate flavored) and ready-made chocolate or vanilla drinks.
www.primenutrition.com.au or Freecall 1800 631 103 (aust)	*Enprocal* powder and *Enprocal Repair* (specially formulated to assist in wound repair) and related products.
www.flavourcreations.com.au or (07)3373 3000 (aust)	*Advital* powder (neutral flavor) whey based, lower in sugar.

INTERNATIONAL SUPPLEMENT PRODUCERS
(some have Australian manufacturing divisions)

www.nestlehealthscience. com.au	*Sustagen Hospital* powder (unflavored, vanilla or chocolate flavor) and *Sustagen* pudding mix. *Resource* drinks (various flavors and formulations) and *Resource Fruit Beverage* (clear juice-style drinks).
www.nutricia.com.au Freecall 1800 060 051 (aust)	*Fortisip* powder (vanilla flavor), *Fortisip* pre-made drinks (various flavours), *Fortijuice* clear, juice style drinks (various flavors) and *Forticreme* (custard-style dessert tubs in various flavors).
www.abbottnutrition.com	*Ensure* powder (vanilla flavor), *Ensure* pre-made drinks (various flavors), *Ensure Pudding* (chocolate, butterscotch or vanilla dessert-style supplements) and *2Cal* high protein supplement.
www.souvenaid.com.au	*Souvenaid* is made by Nutricia but specifically marketed as a brain health supplement.

Whey protein powders and soy based protein powders or other vegan protein powders and drinks are available from health food stores and many online shops. There are too many varieties available to cover them all completely and few contain the added vitamins and minerals that the supplements above do. Check with your dietitian or doctor about these options.

Other resources

Alzheimer's and dementia information and support

Alzheimer's Australia

http://www.fightdementia.org.au

Osteoporosis information and support

Osteoporosis Australia

www.osteoporosis.org.au

www.ingramcontent.com/pod-product-compliance
Lightning Source LLC
Chambersburg PA
CBHW041258040426
42334CB00028BA/3070